The 5-Ounce Gift

A Medical, Philosophical & Spiritual Jewish Guide to Kidney Donation

RABBI DR. SHMULY YANKLOWITZ

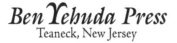

Ben Yehuda Press
Teaneck, New Jersey

Published by Ben Yehuda Press
122 Ayers Court #1B
Teaneck, NJ 07666

http://www.BenYehudaPress.com

To subscribe to our monthly book club and support independent Jewish publishing, visit https://www.patreon.com/BenYehudaPress

Ben Yehuda Press books may be purchased at a discount by synagogues, book clubs, and other institutions buying in bulk. For information, please email: Markets@BenYehudaPress.com

Set in Arno Pro by Raphaël Freeman MISTD, Renana Typesetting

ISBN 13 978-1-953829-24-5

22 23 / 10 9 8 7 6 5 4 3 2 1   20211015

This book is dedicated to my amazing children:

Amiella Rachel
Meir Lev Kook
Maya Neshama
Shaya Or Nafshi Yosef

"My child, when your heart gains
wisdom, my heart rejoices also."

— PROVERBS 23:15

For you, my love knows no bounds.

Along with your beautiful and amazing mother Shoshana, you
are the dearest and most precious gifts in my life. Without you, I
wouldn't be able to do the work I set out to achieve each day. I am
so blessed to be your Abba. You make even the most challenging
days radiate with love and warmth. You reside in my heart, always.

You will have so many opportunities to share your
God-given talents to help others. May you continue
to be brave to accept these opportunities.

For you, my dearest ones, may you each be so blessed to always
find the deepest pearls of wisdom within you, around you,
and wherever you may find them. May they fill you with joy
and delight, all of your long days. I love you with all of me.

Contents

Foreword

Kidney donation is one of the largest ethical problems of our time. So many lives are needlessly lost because of the shortage of donor organs, despite the fact that, in the case of the kidney, donation can be made from a living person as well as at death. There is widespread inertia and ethical negligence about this problem. Many people have not even considered registering as organ donors on death; or, if they have considered it, they may have rejected the idea, believing that such donations are contrary to an ideal they hold about the integrity of the corpse – or even that they are contrary to religious law. And a very tiny minority of people have devoted serious thought to the prospect of donating one of their own kidneys during life, something involving minimal risk to one's health. Still fewer have actually donated. Most of the living donations that do take place go to relatives. So the altruistic donation – giving to a non-relative – is a gift that is rare indeed.

This book, modest in presentation but enormous in importance, aims to change all of this. Rabbi Yanklowitz is himself an altruistic donor. He grabs the reader's attention at the very beginning with a detailed and deeply moving account of the whole process: why he did it, what ethical and religious reflections led him there, what the actual process felt like, what it gave to his recipient. Next, he engages us in philosophical reflection within the Jewish tradition. What are the texts and issues bearing on organ donation, both post mortem and live? How might one argue that a committed Jew should at the very least acknowledge donation as an acceptable moral choice, and at the most, seriously ponder donating as a choice for oneself. Despite my own knowledge of substantial philosophical literature about organ donation, I, though a Jew, knew nothing about what the Jewish tradition says about this topic. I learned effortlessly and with excitement from the book's crystal clear account.

The book goes on to give us historical and current facts about kidney donations, both in the U.S. and in Israel. It then shares other donation stories – including an article by the recipient of Rabbi Yanklowitz's kidney. Finally it describes in detail the work of several important organizations concerned with donation, both here and in Israel. This informational chapter is a terrific idea, because ethics can stimulate thought; but with no source of practical advice, those thoughts might wither away and bear no fruit.

Especially valuable are two interviews conducted by Rabbi Yanklowitz: with Dr. John Fung of the University of Chicago, one of the country's leading transplant surgeons; and with Peter Singer, one of the leading philosophers writing about altruism and our ethical responsibilities. In short, Rabbi Yanklowitz covers all the ground a reader needs to ponder in order to begin a personal process of deliberation.

I know of no book like it. It is moving, uplifting, and profoundly challenging. Although I have no idea how many ounces this book will weigh, it is itself a precious gift!

– Martha C. Nussbaum
The University of Chicago

Acknowledgements

One does not acquire Jewish wisdom lightly. Pursuing it takes a lifetime of rigorous study, and requires perspicacity and open-heartedness; it helps, too, if one is blessed with understanding guides and wise teachers. That lifetime of study should not be viewed as a means to achieve intellectual glory. Rather, studying Jewish texts is a journey with infinite steps and no end in sight, a pleasurable pursuit for its own sake.

The opportunity to study and to write about the material in this book has been a delight. In all my years as a Jewish educator, I've never encountered ideas or emotions quite like the ones I explore in this book. It was both a challenging and illuminating experience to approach these ancient ideas and to apply them to this very particular moral challenge. It is truly a revelatory encounter with the timeless totality of Jewish wisdom.

The book you hold in your hands was perhaps my most difficult one to write to date. Many partners made this book possible. I would like to start by saying how grateful I am to Larry Yudelson of Ben Yehuda Press for his empathetic vision to help me to bring this book into print, and to editor Laura Logan for her thoughtful and thorough editing of the manuscript.

I'm also very grateful to colleagues, teachers, and friends such as Rabbi Eliezer Finkelman, Rabbi Avram Herzog, Abraham J. Frost, Dr. John Fung, Judry Subar, and Emma Offenberg for their support and contributions. I am so grateful for your hard work throughout the years. Thank you all so much for your attentiveness to this work. The assistance from these esteemed colleagues was invaluable as I made my way through my spiritual and intellectual journey.

I am forever grateful to Menachem Friedman at Renewal for holding my hand through my journey, to Dr. Edward Chinn and the amazing medical team at Mt. Sinai Hospital.

Most importantly, this book wouldn't have been possible without the everlasting love of my beautiful and brilliant wife Shoshana and our wonderful children, Amiella, Lev, Maya, and Shay. Whenever I found myself in need of inspiration, I thought of my family. Thank you for all the joy and light you share with me every day. I love you with all my heart!

Introduction

I always wanted to do something big with my life.

I learned quickly that, despite many attempts, I would never become a world-famous scientist, a disrupting inventor, a virtuoso musician, or the President of the United States – mainly for lack of talent but also because I didn't want to chase an empty vessel of celebrity or fame. I wanted to focus my life on another goal: the goal of alleviating suffering.

This basic framework, while elementary, also grounded me in an ideal I knew that I could follow. I reflected on the famous adage from the Talmud that states that one who saves a life is akin to saving the entire world. Yet, I also realized that I never wanted my profession to be that of a police officer, a soldier, a surgeon, or a fireman. So how would I get a chance to alleviate another person's pain and woe? Maybe one day I'd be at the scene when someone was drowning or being attacked, and I could intervene? Maybe there'd be a circumstance where I'd perform CPR on someone? Or enter a burning building to save a family? Grandiose visions, for sure. But I couldn't rely on these improbable scenarios formulated in my imagination.

But then, I stumbled across another way to save a life, one where I *knew* I could actually be of service to someone else. I heard about living kidney donation, and it startled my soul. I don't recall the exact moment, but a series of such moments opened me to the dream of saving a life. And then questions formed in my mind: Is it possible? Is it safe? Would I, could I, actually save a life?

I remember being sure never to raise the idea with my parents until later in the process. I was already an adult when I decided to think about the procedure seriously, but I wasn't ready yet to approach them for their advice and counsel. When I finally told them, they responded as expected, as virtually every parent would: they attempted to discourage me. Vigorously. (Strangely enough, if my children approached me with this desire, I'd probably try to dissuade them too. Maybe it's in our parental DNA?)

Years later, when I raised the issue again with my wife, I didn't go the route I had with my parents. Rather, I avoided the straightforward question of donation and instead raised the idea of being tested. My wife Shoshana told me later that she knew what I was really asking. And, on some cosmic plane, we both knew deep down that if testing allowed me to donate, I would almost certainly end up doing it. We knew there would be hundreds of little barriers – tests, logistics, research, conversation, and prayer – but that my stubborn conviction would push through those.

How could it not? I'd spent years teaching around the country on the topic of alleviating suffering and the limitless value of saving life. I'd talked about the significance of sacrifice and of actualizing our life potential by elevating others. I would ask questions about the required extent of our financial sacrifice in order to save another. I would explore our obligations to the sick and the vulnerable on an individual and communal level. If I expected others to behave in a way that I would not, might my words, to some extent, be hollow and hypocritical?

I pondered and meditated deeply on the task at hand.

As I pondered, I thought about my father's poignant pushback: What if I could spend my energy saving thousands by advocating for this issue rather than put my life and health at risk? I considered this option. But, in my mind, I thought back to Gandhi and how he would not tell a little boy to stop eating sugar as the boy's mother requested until he himself stopped eating sugar. I knew that if I were going to try to change the system and promote the dream of no one dying from kidney failure that I would need to live this experience, and donate a kidney, myself.

The questions I considered before undergoing my kidney donation journey were not only practical but also moral and theological. Did I believe myself to be the true owner of my body? Did God put a backup kidney in me *for me*, or for someone else?

Many potential living kidney donors don't consider the question unless they are asked by a sick family member, friend, or community member. That wasn't my case. Rather, as one engaged in the study of moral philosophy and religion, it was a theoretical question: Can I? Should I? Must I?

In the end, I was motivated by a mix of faith and philosophy. I got myself into trouble when teaching, and taking two stories I shared to heart:

The first was from Professor Peter Singer, the radical utilitarian who argued that people have a moral responsibility to sacrifice luxuries for the sake of saving a life. If a second kidney was unlikely to be needed to live a full, robust life, how could one justify letting another die while keeping one's luxury organ?[1]

The second was a story about a Holocaust survivor who –

---

1. Professor Singer would later disagree with me that having two kidneys constitutes the notion that one of them is a luxury rather than a biological reality. See our interview later in this book.

after going through so much trauma himself – saved his son who struggled from renal failure.

Then there were all the textual ideas I came across that led me to ask big questions. I felt that if I were not to achieve much with my life, perhaps the recipient of my second kidney would achieve something great with his or her second chance at life. I was motivated by a rather intense and graphic passage written by Nahmanides:[2]

> God commanded that when a person sins, he must bring a sacrifice, rest his hands upon it, corresponding to actions, and offer verbal confession, corresponding to speech. He must burn in fire the innards and kidneys, which are the instruments of thought and desire, and the legs, corresponding to man's arms and legs which do all of his work. And he must burn the blood on the altar, corresponding to his own blood, so that when he does all these things, he should think that he had sinned to his God with his body and soul, and it would [therefore] be fitting for him to pour his own blood and burn his own body, were it not for the Creator's loving kindness, who accepted a substitution from him. This sacrifice atones [for him], its blood instead of his own blood, a soul instead of his soul, the primary organs of the sacrifice corresponding to his own organs.[3]

I felt that my kidney could be my *korban* (sacrificial offering). I owe my entire body and existence to God, and I wanted to repay an enormous debt. At some primal level, I hoped that this donation could be a sort of *tikkun* (repair) for my past mistakes.

---

2. 13th century, Spain and Israel. Nahmanides is also known as Ramban, an acronym for his full name, Rabbi Moshe ben Nahman.

3. Nahmanides commentary on Leviticus 1:8

A question plagued me: "What if I end up taking more from this world than I give back?" I was sure that, up until that point, I had taken more from the world than I had given. Consider just the first years of life: others carrying me and changing my diapers. Then I sat in classrooms while others taught me. It would take over two decades to even enter the workforce in any meaningful way. What had I really given?

There were naturally many pressures not to donate. Many of my friends tried to dissuade me. One friend told me, "Surgeons make a lot of money and aren't really motivated by saving lives." I was not dissuaded. First, I felt that it was not my place to judge another's motives, especially when they are doing good. Second, why should I care how much a surgeon is paid? In truth, surgery is a complex talent that few are capable of and I felt that experts should indeed be well compensated. But other questions plagued me as well:

What about *my* kids and family?

What about the risks?

What if *I* need a kidney at some point in the future?

What about the pain? I'm not one of those pain-resistant types, nor am I a risk-taker with my body.

Still, and perhaps because of the above questions, I remember that once my heart was convinced of what to do, I emotionally struggled to pursue my path. Panic filled me. I woke up sweating in the night. I had trouble focusing at work. I had trouble looking my children in the eyes when I considered the path ahead. I knew it was my path, but I also knew there were risks, fears, and aversions that I would need to overcome. I've never been anything like a purely spiritual guru living with peaceful equanimity: rather, I'd also been plagued in the past with anxious feelings and deep fears and knew they would come to fore here as well.

The remarkable people in this story were the researchers and medical teams that made organ donation possible. My hero was my wife Shoshana, who made everything possible for me. I just laid myself on the table and went to sleep while they opened me up. Then I mostly relaxed and recovered. I had it easy. My precious wife, on the other hand, stayed at the hospital with me, and took care of me and our babies with enormous capability, grace, and love, all with a smile and without complaining once. What she did, and how she did it, was truly remarkable. Heaven will testify that, in fact, she was the one who saved a life.

Throughout my kidney donation journey, I recall having few resources available to me. Which doctors could I talk to? Which past donors could I grill about their experience? Which mental health professionals could support me? This book, which has stirred inside my mind for many years, is intended to be a modest contribution for those exploring this journey and for those who want to learn more about the process from someone who experienced it.

But let me be clear about what this book is and what it is not.

I am not a doctor, and this isn't a book about modern medicine. This book is not a substitute for talking with medical professionals. Yes, while I have done an enormous amount of medical research and interviews with doctors and those working in the field, you can and should go forward with the procedure only after reaching your own personal conclusions based upon your own research and conversations. Godspeed to you.

The book that you now hold in your hands is about my journey, but be warned that it is not an authoritative account of kidney donation in any aggregate sense. Dear reader, instead, I promise to provide to you the many elements that went into *my* organ donation: How did I decide? What was my concrete experience within testing, surgery, and recovery? What have others' experiences (with whom I spoke or researched) looked like? What are some of the moral, political, economic, and medical calculations involved in the global situation today? How does the Jewish tradition understand the ethical issues related to organ donation?

This book is about my journey. It's about that personal, inner journey (through philosophy, theology, and soul searching). It's about an activist journey (how to create deeper change to save more lives). It's about a medical journey (through researching the data intellectually and internalizing the data emotionally). It's about a Jewish journey (through texts and traditions and timeless Jewish wisdom). It's also about journeys of other donors, Jewish educators, and Jewish leaders. We'll explore organizations that support Jewish organ donation. We'll explore organ donation as seen by a transplant surgeon.

This book is not only for those considering kidney donation. It is also for those supporting others in need of a transplant or supporting others who are in the process of donating. It is for rabbis and other clergy supporting community members in this spiritual journey. It is for those interested in Jewish texts and moral dilemmas.

I'm not here to attempt to convince you or any reader to donate his or her kidney. This is, of course, a deeply personal journey with so many factors to consider. I reflect here upon my experience and the experience of others in order that many will be able in turn to fully consider this path; but people will have to navigate through their own moral, spiritual, and familial deliberations. Follow this path, or don't. But still, come with me as we explore the many dimensions of altruistic[4] kidney donation and all the possibilities it gives to others who seek a new lease on life.

---

4. Altruistic living donation is the term for when one gives to a stranger instead of giving to a family member or a friend.

Unlike any other issue I'm involved with, on this particular issue I make my readers a rare offer. To anyone who is considering kidney donation, who has read this book, I will offer my time on the phone to provide any support I can. I have been blessed to watch my brother-in-law donate his kidney to my father-in-law and to talk with countless others who have grappled and ultimately donated. I've learned a lot about how others think about pain, risk, connectedness, and responsibility. One donor told me that he considers the act "heroic." Others said, "it's really not such a big deal." I assure you that my goal is not to convince, but merely to be a friend and guide through the experience. I find such calls and conversations deeply rewarding.

NOTE: All references and resources cited in this book were accurate at the time of publication.

Chapter 1

My Story

Making the Decision

I always wanted to save a life. I prepared for moments of crisis that could arise and how I would act. But those moments never came. No one landed on my doorstep. I wasn't equipped to become a surgeon or a firefighter or a soldier. But then it occurred to me that I needed to be more proactive: I realized that there were people dying right now of something I could directly help with. As soon as I realized this, I felt a pain in my gut. It was as if it was now totally clear to me what I would have to do. I couldn't imagine any ideas emerging that could come to contradict what I now knew so deeply.

Nonetheless, for some years, I silenced the thought. I was young, I was on a journey, and I was running. The faster I could run in work, in life, the less I would have to reflect on the issue of cruel treatment of animals, knowing that eventually I would have to become a vegan. Or, when researching orphans, knowing one day I would have to foster or adopt.

What does it mean to take a risk?

It is not as rare as one might think that people risk their lives for a higher purpose. Consider those who enlist in the military or in the police force or in the fire department. They are not extremists but individuals driven by meaning, by a purpose, by a belief in saving life even if there are real risks. Are those who run into burning houses to rescue victims insane? Or are they heroes who believe in the infinite value of human life? How about women who spend nine months (plus recovery time) developing a child within their womb, giving their bodies much stress, and then suffering pangs while giving birth?[1] Are they extremists to undergo such treatment and procedures? It is hard to make such decisions about accepting risks to life, but it is also rewarding. Do I regret donating a kidney? I only regret that I can't do it again!

Some suggested that I should keep both of my kidneys, thus keeping a kidney in reserve in case I, or a family member, were to need it. However, it seemed more likely that I might keep the kidney, only to waste it, without it helping me or anyone else. If I had a life jacket on a perfectly working boat, would I not throw it to someone drowning in the water – rather than hold on to it just in case I might need it at some point? That would be a morally absurd choice. I also now know, as a past donor, that I would have more resources to find another donor if needed for me or a family member in the future.

I wondered if it might make more sense to just save my kidneys for after death, to be donated at that time.[2] But I learned that it is generally considered medically better to receive a

---

1. The World Health Organization reported in 2014 that the mortality rate for those giving birth was about 3 out of 10,000. Interestingly enough, this is statistically the same as the risk to someone donating a kidney. In both cases, one gives the gift of life and accepts risks, modest but real, along the way. The risk is only slightly higher for automobile accidents. Should one not drive due to the risks?

2. Contrary to common perception, donating organs after death is permitted by Jewish law, with the proviso that measures are taken to keep the body intact and otherwise treated with respect.

kidney from a living donor than from a cadaver. First, the kidney will most often be younger and healthier. Research has shown that kidneys from deceased donors tend not to last as long as kidneys from living donors. Second, removing kidneys from cadavers presents problems. In some cases, the kidney could perhaps be removed too soon, when, from a Jewish law perspective, the donor may not yet be legally "dead." In other cases, the kidney may perhaps be removed so late that it is no longer usable.

Further, the Centers for Disease Control and Prevention reports that nearly three million people die each year in America. Of these, I learned, only about two percent have organs that could be harvested, and only about half of those die in a such a way that donation could take place.

But how would I feel if I were to die younger because of this donation? Would it have been worth it? It is hard to sustain that scary thought in my heart.

Conversations with parents can be the most challenging. Even adults can sometimes become like young children again when inviting parents into major life decisions. Adult children might want approval but not advice, but it seems unfair to expect that approval to be immediate. If the decision took you years of research and thought, why would you expect a loved one to approve immediately? For this reason, one considering this should prepare for pushback. Further, one cannot expect – and maybe would not welcome – a dispassionate response from a spouse, parent, or child who loves you.

For these reasons, I suggest you consider revealing your interest in the process in advance, long before declaring your decision. Give your family time to adjust to the coming decision. Simply sharing the final decision will almost inevitably receive pushback.

For myself, I knew that if I ever needed a kidney, I would

be in a better position after donating. Because kidney disease typically attacks both kidneys, not just one, if I were to have such a disease, I would have needed a new kidney anyway. But as a past donor, I would be bumped to the top of the list rather than waiting at the bottom. So, one might suggest that I was better off – and even looking after my own welfare – after donating.

The world was changing all around me at the time. With the passing of the Affordable Care Act, health insurance companies could no longer block coverage for those with preexisting conditions. This helps to protect donors. However, while healthcare costs are covered during the transplant, it is important to note that if long-term health problems emerge, the transplant center will not cover those. For this reason, some transplant centers will not accept donors who don't have health insurance to protect them in the long-term. The Affordable Care Act makes it easier for the centers in question to accept such donors.

Is it wrong to choose to whom to donate? At first, I didn't know the answer to such a question. Is it "playing God" to decide to donate to this person instead of that person? I decided it was not a problem at all, and I realized that the moral tension of trying to decide is healthy. If one chooses to donate to a family member, that is praiseworthy. If a black woman really wants to donate to a black woman, that is praiseworthy. If someone only wants to donate to a child instead of an adult, that is praiseworthy. If a Jew wants to donate to a Jew or specifically to a gentile, either choice is praiseworthy as well. I recently posted publicly about a Muslim little boy who needed a liver donation and I was flooded with Muslim volunteers and questions from Muslim Americans around the country. No one should judge or critique one's individual choice. Of course, on the collective systems level, there should be no discrimination on who receives a kidney. But ultimately it is only up to a donor to decide, just as donors decide where they wish to give financial donations.

Stated in negative terms – if a white person would say, "I will not give to a person of color" or a man would say, "I will not give to a woman" – those preferences seem racist (and, in the second case, chauvinistic). State the preferences in positive terms, and perhaps they do not seem tainted. The person who says, "I wish to give to a person like me" has at least decided to donate. Giving to "a person like me" certainly involves more generosity than not giving at all. In practice, most donations today are not purely "altruistic," in that most donors exercise some discretion in the choice of recipient. If we reject donations from those who want to influence the choice of the recipient, then our quest for purity of motive will result in saving fewer lives.

I concluded that it is okay, even good, to give to someone in an identity group that one most closely identifies with. Jews can and perhaps should donate to Jews. African Americans can and should be encouraged to donate to African Americans. It is great to go beyond one's identity or values community, but it is also great to give within. It is not wrong to donate to a child or an adult, to a neighbor or to someone on the other side of the world, to a stranger or a friend.

We must be gentler with ourselves. Saving a life is saving a life and we should all embrace the opportunity that is presented to us or that feels right to us. We certainly shouldn't let others who haven't donated judge the way in which we have done so.

One can start "a chain" of giving. It works like this: Sarah has blood type A, so she can't donate to her dad, who has blood type O. Sarah donates to Jim's mom who has type A, in exchange for Jim donating to Sarah's dad, since he has type O blood. Sometimes the chain can be super long; the longest to date involved over 100 donations!

I received mixed advice about starting a chain, since the chain might grow to include many steps, and the process could therefore involve complex coordination, which would take time and thereby delay the donation. Once I knew who my recipient was, I didn't feel that I could make him wait any longer.

For me, I was inspired by the mitzvah of *"lo ta'amod al dam rei'echa"* ("do not stand idly by the blood of your fellow")[3] and by the mitzvah of *piku'ah nefesh* (saving a life).[4] I couldn't imagine living any longer with the luxury of a spare kidney (unlikely to be needed) knowing that someone else would definitely die if I didn't donate. I knew there would be pain, risks, and some recovery, but I want, and strive, to give as much of myself as I can to our local community, to the global Jewish community, and to the world. I recall my wife, Shoshana, saying, as she herself was considering donating her kidney, that perhaps God would be less likely to take her early to get her parts if she had given them already.[5]

In the end, I felt I needed to heed the Torah's call of *"uvaharta bahayim"* ("choose life!")[6] and *"v'ahavta l'rei'acha kamocha"* ("you shall love your fellow as yourself").[7] I couldn't stop thinking that I can't imagine a world where I would need saving and no one would do it for me. How unloved I would feel in a selfish world. I couldn't imagine a world where we just stood idly by. Could this be what it means to bring a *korban* (a humble offering) in our time? Could this be what it means for Am Yisrael (the Nation of Israel) to be *"ish ehad b'leiv ehad"* ("one person with one heart")?[8]

---

3. Leviticus 19:16
4. Babylonian Talmud Shabbat 150a
5. She was naturally being characteristically humble with such a thought, since she lives a life deeply committed to service and kindness.
6. Deuteronomy 30:19
7. Leviticus 19:18
8. The comment of Rashi (11th century, France) on Exodus 19:2. Rashi

As I opened my heart to this mitzvah, I started to hear miracle stories. I heard that the wife of a brain surgeon, who was struggling for a long time with kidney failure, put up *mezuzot* on their doorposts (they were atheists!) and the next day they got the call that the donor was found for him. They then learned that the words *mezuzot* and *kelayot* (kidneys) have the same *gematria* (numerical value of the Hebrew letters)! We need not embrace a full confidence in *gematria* to find this story amazing.[9]

Testing

For me, the first stage of testing simply included a blood test and a urine test. Later testing included more blood tests, twenty-four hours of urine collection, an EKG, a CAT scan, an ultrasound, conversations with nurses and nephrologists, a transplant coordinator, mental health professionals, and so many more.

I recall so clearly spending those two days of testing and preparation in NYC at Mt. Sinai Hospital. I was exhausted, to say the least. I found the team to be sensitive, patient, honest, and informed. I appreciated that they were trying neither to persuade nor dissuade me regarding my decision to donate my kidney. They appreciated the complexity of the situation.

The medical team told me that there was an error in the assessment of my 24-hour urine collection. I couldn't believe it. I joked with my wife that it would be a lot of fun to carry a urine bucket around with me for a day again. It would make for good professional advancement!

I also found the hospital to be extremely protective of

---

is among the earliest and most prolific of the medieval commentators on the Torah.

9. My friend, a Modern Orthodox rabbi living in New York who wishes to remain anonymous, was the donor who told me this story.

donors. Although the hospital personnel have a profit incentive in maximizing transplants, they also know how much is at stake with their reputation and licenses if anyone were to be suspected of any form of coercion. So, after every medical exam, I also had countless conversations with doctors, psychologists, social workers, and donor advocates assessing my motives and mental fitness to donate.

After one has undergone blood test matching, it is not over. The medical team must do cross-matching. Here the blood cells of the recipient and the blood cells of the donor are combined to see how they react together. In a positive match, they exist alongside each other without causing trouble. In a negative match, the blood cells of the recipient attack the blood cells from the donor, indicating that the transplant would cause trouble. It is not all black and white, as there can be a range of intermediate reactions. Recipients usually have to take anti-rejection medication for the rest of their lives to ensure the continued coexistence.

All of the tests and evaluations are free and covered by the transplant center or by the recipient's insurance. A side benefit: These elaborative examinations can benefit the potential donor, since they can detect problems that the donor would not have otherwise suspected. Early detection and prompt treatment can save the potential donor's life!

My biggest challenge during the testing was the MRI. It was my first time, and I wasn't prepared. It was just me alone in the tube for 40 minutes, unable to move. I felt trapped, claustrophobic, lost, and scared. I was challenged to cultivate a new level of faith. I would not seek for Divine intervention but Divine intimacy to help me get through my time stuck in the tube.

When I was 7 or 8 years old, I was mistakenly taken to see a film called "Fire in the Sky." It was a horror film about a man abducted by aliens. I ran out crying and it haunted me for years. In truth, the MRI experience was the first time I was brought back to that film. I started to feel as though I was abducted by aliens and trapped. Who would rescue me? I didn't "squeeze the ball" (notifying the staff that I needed to come out) because I knew that I needed to meet this challenge of completing the task, but I was in great anguish.

In the testing stage, I started to grapple with the question of whether I should make my exploratory journey public or keep it private. I struggled with whether to share my thought process and experiences. On the one hand, giving anonymously is a great Jewish value. An anonymous donor does not look for credit or reward. On the other hand, going public demonstrates a value, too, as it encourages others to engage in the mitzvah as well.

I decided that I would be public but work to be as modest and unpersuasive as possible. I would use "I" experiential language and not "we should" or "we must" language. Kidney donation is very personal and not for everyone.

I felt that I wanted to approach this issue, like most, with an activist spirit. Currently, for most people, donating a kidney has no place on their personal agenda. How could we campaign to inspire individuals to at least consider this lifesaving mitzvah?

I experienced a deep personal transformation in testing my limits regarding how much I was willing to give. Knowing that there were over 4 million people around the world waiting for a kidney transplant, what would it mean to give to only one? I hoped that by teaching and writing about the subject, I would be able to help more than one person. I knew I could be a stronger and wiser advocate for saving life after going through the transplant myself. Indeed, since I chose to be public about my journey, countless people have asked to meet, called, and emailed with questions, as they consider (and in many cases pursue) this journey for themselves.

Even once the testing was complete and I was cleared, I still felt a major weight hanging over my head. As I mentioned earlier in this book, I began to wonder why I should go to so much trouble just to save one life? Might I be more effective by advocating to save many lives and not have to go through surgery? I kept recalling that the Talmud teaches: "Whoever saves one life is considered as having saved the entire world."[10]

Pre-Surgery

The morning leading into the surgery was very spiritual. All the testing and analysis had been completed. I knew I had already made the decision. Now, I just needed to experience the day fully, emotionally and spiritually. Right when I woke up, I went to the *mikveh* (the Jewish spiritual bath) to try to bring a purity of intentions to the door. I was told by a previous donor, a Hasidic rabbi, that Rabbi Binyamin Eisenberger's advice for kidney donors was to go to the *mikveh* the morning of a surgery and then recite the biblical account of the *Akeidat Yitzhak* (Binding of Isaac, Genesis 22) three times after *shaharit* (morning prayers).[11] So I did that and then recited some Tehillim (Psalms). My friend, a psychiatrist and spiritual healer, had recorded a meditation for me to listen to in the car. It was a deeply meditative and prayerful morning.

My beloved wife Shoshana drove me to the hospital and

---

10. Mishnah Sanhedrin 4:5; incidentally, the same sentence appears later in the Quran 5:32.

11. I was very emotional reading the *Akeidah* that morning. And I felt so relieved at the moment when God released Abraham from the obligation to sacrifice his son. I hoped, in some way, that maybe I was able to offer my kidney in place of some greater sacrifice.

stayed by my side the whole morning. Reflecting back on the morning at the hospital leading up to the surgery, I can still feel how intense and raw my emotions were that morning. The emotional highlight of the morning was meeting Yossi, the recipient, right before the surgery. I was already in my pre-op gown. When he walked into my room, I knew immediately, from the picture, who he was. I ran over and hugged him. He held me so tight and we both sobbed. We told each other we loved each other. We had never met or talked, but I instantly felt connected to him. Our fates were now intertwined.

In pre-op, they gave me my IV and prepared me for surgery. Everything was new to me in the experience: the hospital gown, the feeling of the IV, the culture of the room, and more. Before being wheeled out, I placed my *tzitzit* (Jewish fringed garment) under my pillow to feel closeness to God and in the hope of some Divine protection.

Never before had I felt so grateful for the mitzvah of *tzitzit*. When I entered surgery, the surgeon would, of course, not let me wear them. But he let me place them under my operating table pillow. They reminded me of my spiritual purpose and my desire for closeness with the One who sustains life. I thought of them and planned to recite the *Shema*[12] prayer as the last words from my lips before having my body opened. Fear reminds us that we are alive and vulnerable; putting on a front of imperturbability is absurd. Buber was right: "In telling a lie, the spirit commits treason against itself."[13] More than 80 times in the Torah, G-d reminds us not to fear, knowing how pervasive and destructive an emotion of existential paralysis can be. My *tallit* (the technical name for the garment on which

---

12. The Shema is the Jewish prayer, traditionally recited twice daily, acknowledging God's oneness and presence in our lives.
13. *Good and Evil*, 7.

the *tzitzit* fringes are placed) shall give me, I felt, wings to fly[14] from despair to liberation. I felt the sentiment of the verse, "I fear no evil, for You are with me" (Psalm 23).

My wife, Shoshana, was with me all the way up to the point where they pushed me from pre-op to the operating room. I teared up yet again as the medical professionals wheeled me away. I raised up my hand, thumb toward the ceiling, once I could no longer see her. I did this in solidarity and in faith to reassure her that all was going to be okay. But, as I tried to remain strong, I cried knowing that this could in fact be the last time I would ever see her again.

Once in the operating room, the anesthesiologist placed a mask over my mouth and I recall, in a remarkably surreal and spiritual experience, reciting the *Shema* up until the point that I was knocked out. The surgery lasted about 3–4 hours.

I knew it was my left kidney that was to be removed. Most typically the left kidney is optimal since there are longer blood vessels which lead to easier attachment in the recipient and since the liver is not in the way. The surgery I had was a "laparoscopic left donor nephrectomy." The surgeons made five incisions: four on the side for the cameras ("laparoscopic" means using fiber optic cables to enable cameras), and one bigger incision, about three inches, in front, to remove the kidney. Later, I read the report of the dozens of tasks that took place during the surgery and I was amazed at how much had happened. I was also startled to read that there was some excess bleeding and that they used surgical staples to stop that. My amazing surgeon, Dr. Edward Chinn said this whole procedure I underwent was the standard, normal procedure, the same as other surgeons would have performed.

---

14. It is fascinating that the Hebrew word *kanaf* means both wing and corner, and is in fact the word used in the Torah in describing where on the garment the *tzitzit* are to be placed.

Post-Surgery

I don't remember waking up. My first memory was on my way from my recovery room to my hospital room, when I was reunited with my wife. Indeed, she was the first face I recall seeing and it brought me so much joy that, with my first words, I blurted out: "You got more beautiful!" I spoke the simple truth I felt so deeply, but the loopy feeling from the anesthesia helped me to say it more immediately and fervently.

I then recall reciting the *berachah* (blessing) *"oseh maaseh bereishit"* (thanking God for the miracles of life and creation).[15] Returning to consciousness, I recall feeling that I was being brought back to life. It wasn't at all like waking up in the morning. It was far more surreal: like being born, but as an adult.[16]

Shoshana reminds me, although I don't recall this, that as I was being wheeled around the hospital, I would give blessings to everyone we would see, very intensely.

Within minutes of my kidney being placed within Yossi, the doctors witnessed it aiding the process of healthy urination, a crucial sign of acceptance and success. To me, hearing this news was nothing less than miraculous. God had placed a kidney within me for him, and now it was home!

In terms of pain tolerance, I'm probably average. I'm not someone who can easily handle a lot of pain but also not super intolerant to pain. I probably lean more toward the weaker side than the pain-tolerant side. One sign of that is that I always maxed out my pain meds in the hospital. I recall being upset with one nurse practitioner who wouldn't give me more when I requested them (he's a friend now). But I got off pain meds relatively quickly once I left the hospital. While in the hospital, getting out of bed was the hardest for me.

---

15. This *berachah* literally praises God "Who performs the act of creation."
16. Perhaps this is similar to the "birth" of Adam and Eve, born as adults.

I was blessed with visitors. My wife and children visited. Some of my rabbis and friends came by to pray and sing together. A Hasidic rabbi, a former kidney donor and now a dear friend, came by in the middle of the night to watch over me, laying upon the guest bench. Children from the Satmar Bikkur Cholim came by to bring me snacks. Each visitor and each visit from a medical professional made me feel less alone and brought me comfort.

Recovery
But how would I recover?

When I left the hospital (after 3 days, 2 nights), I recall being pushed out in a wheelchair. I couldn't believe how profoundly healing the sunlight was. It was also startling, as I was shell-shocked from the intensity of the experience.

My wife and children were staying at my in-laws' home. I decided that I didn't want to sleep at my in-laws' since it would be noisy with lots of family, especially from my little children. So, I decided to go to a hotel for 4–5 nights. This turned out to be a difficult time because I didn't welcome the isolation and lack of support. I recall crying in my bed at night, sweating through all my clothes, finding frustrations with urination, swelling, pain, being bloated, and from the isolation without help.

A highlight of my stay at the hotel came when Shoshana and my kids would briefly visit. It would light up my world. The other highlight came when two Hasidic singers came by to perform for me and sing with me. That brought such a deep joy.

After the week passed and Shoshana picked me up to go to her parents' house in Teaneck, New Jersey, it was the first time I experienced the sunlight since leaving the hospital. I recall feeling such immense joy that that week had closed and that I was miraculously now on my way to recovery.

It was never a cakewalk for me, but each day things got easier. I spent the second week in bed but with increasing comfort.

During the third and fourth weeks I was able to work and just move around the house slowly. By four weeks, I was excited that I could pick up my babies again. And I was ready for life as usual again. Thank God, I never had any complications or significant discomforts after that 4-week mark.

Everyone's recovery will be different. The donor, post-op, can typically be out of bed on day two and walking around. Typically, one should allow for the first two weeks to completely rest, and 4–6 weeks for any strenuous activity. I personally started working from bed after two weeks but wasn't 100% until 4 weeks.

Most donors only stay in the hospital for two nights, but in some cases the hospital will allow, or even encourage, 3–4 nights. In more extreme cases, it could be up 7 nights. In my case, I only stayed for two. I requested to stay for an extra night since I appreciated the monitoring and support but, for some reason, they denied my request, deeming me fit to leave.

The donor, post-op, will need to wait a few weeks to start driving again, swimming (or immersing fully in a bath), and at least four weeks before lifting anything heavy (even a child). Unless one develops infections – always a concern – the donor should be going at full speed by six weeks at the latest. Of course, one's age and general health will affect the timing and duration of recovery.

While recovering, it is important to rest, walk, and keep your spirits up. It's important for the donor to establish a support system for various needs. You can fall into depression after any major surgery, especially if you're used to being busy and connected, and then suddenly find yourself confined to a bed and more socially isolated than usual. It's also important to use your spirometer[17] (an apparatus which measures the

---

17. This should be given to a donor at the hospital and one can bring it home with them.

movement of air in and out of the lungs) to keep your lungs clear and to avoid breathing problems such as pneumonia.

For managing pain, at some point, you switch from morphine to oral narcotics and then you can switch from narcotics (like codeine) to just Tylenol. You might need anti-nausea medications while recovering from the anesthesia and while on the more intense post-op pain meds. You may also need stool softeners and laxatives to aid digestion.[18]

Emotions before the surgery, after the surgery, and years later, will be different for everyone. For me, at different times I felt pride, fulfillment, fear, anxiety, joy, and just total emotional overload. It was one of the most intense experiences of my life. I recall crying so many times, which is not usual for me. My most vivid memory was leaving the hotel where I had stayed alone for a few days after being discharged from the hospital.[19] Walking outside and feeling the fresh sunlight on my face, and taking that first deep breath of fresh air, I found myself bawling at something so simple that I normally took for granted.

The scars serve as reminders to me of my human frailty and of this spiritual journey.

I wasn't only nervous about the risks, but also about the experience itself. One aspect of the surgery I was most nervous about was the breathing tube. I had witnessed my father in a complication after open-heart surgery struggling with a breathing tube in his mouth, and I was concerned about what appeared to be a traumatic and invasive experience. As it happened, the tube was put in only after I was asleep and was taken out before I woke up; I had no pain or discomfort in my

---

18. Morphine can lead to constipation.
19. Many in recovery prefer to have company and care. I preferred to have total quiet and isolation. I don't know if I made the right choice. I mainly feared seeing my little children but not being able to adequately engage with them.

throat at all. Another concern I had was the urinary catheter, which was going to be a new experience for me. But that too was put in when I was asleep and the removal a day or two after surgery was not uncomfortable or as embarrassing as I imagined it would be; it took only seconds. For the next day or two, I mostly urinated into a bottle. I recall waiting for a nurse to replace my urine bucket and feeling so humbled by the sense of basic dependency on others.

Two weeks after the surgery, I visited the surgeon so that he could review the incisions to ensure all looked okay.

I took some time off work after the surgery. While some federal employees may find that they're granted thirty days off to recover, state policies will differ. I believe that all donors should be granted paid leave. No one should have to jeopardize their job security or salary for donating.

What kind of a life would I be able to live after donating? The only two activities I was told to refrain from long-term were competitive boxing and using ibuprofen (the active ingredient in Advil or Motrin).[20] Donating a kidney has actually led me to living a healthier lifestyle, being more aware of the needs of my body. I've become more mindful of remaining hydrated and of the importance of a healthy diet and consistent exercise. It's important to have an annual check on your creatine levels[21] and blood pressure.

After my surgery, I wasn't concerned only with my recovery but with how my recipient was doing. After the surgery, Yossi, my recipient, emailed me this (translated from the Hebrew):

---

20. A donor is typically advised to limit or completely avoid NSAIDS (non-steroidal anti-inflammatory drugs) since they alter the blood flow, which can affect one's kidney. One is typically advised to use acetaminophen (like Tylenol) for pain relief instead.
21. Creatine is an amino acid located in the muscles and is an important source of energy.

Shmuly, how are you?

After the surgery, I did not stop to ask if you're okay. It was important to me, [but] I was scared a little.

So, first of all I desire your well-being; I will always ask for you to get stronger, to get well soon, and to feel good.

What you did for me is the rare humane act, an act that a normal person does not think about at all; those who think to do something like that probably have special powers, great faith, a lot of love, and a strong desire to help and save lives.

I did not believe there are such people, and today I still do not digest that a person who does not know me from across the world, heard my story and wanted to save my life.

Today I know that because of you, thanks to the desire, concern, sensitivity and your belief, today I got a new life from you, a life I had forgotten (even with dialysis).

What is more beautiful, exciting, powerful and strong is that God gave us life – but also gave us humans the ability to give life to each other.

I believe that things do not happen by chance; I believe that, even though people cannot relate to the causes. I also believe that things that happen bring us to other stages in life, teach us something, and change us for the better.

I believe we live here in this world to experience good experiences and less good experiences, powerful enough to remind us that we are human beings here in this world together to help each other.

I still do not [fully] digest and feel the dream, but I know it happened and I know it probably had to happen for good things to happen afterwards.

And now when the pain begins to pass slowly, I can see it as a kind of an experience, powerful and very strong, between two people, one who wanted to save the other who got saved. From here the two of us just grow and evolve to become better people, stronger, full of faith, to encounter good things and good people – there are quite a few.

I always wanted a brother since I was a kid; I always wanted [one], and now after we are connected by blood, I can say that this dream has come true and I have a new brother.

I would love to meet you and stay in touch.

"Thanks" is this little word, or in fact such a big word; if it were bigger, then I'd tell you the same in the bigger word.

A big and huge thank you!!!

Joseph Azran

I accepted his invitation to be family now – indeed, we always will be.

After I finally made it to *shul*[22] after my recovery, I *bentched gomel* (the commonly used Yiddish term for reciting the blessing formally thanking God for surviving),[23] and each year I continue to thank God for the miracle.

---

22. the synagogue

23. This prayer is recited in public by those who have survived a dangerous experience. In full it reads: "Blessed is God, King of the universe, who brings to the undeserving good outcomes."

Chapter 2

The Mitzvah to Save a Life

Saving a Life

Here we will explore some of the Jewish foundation texts dealing with various moral concerns involved with taking risk to help others. As with most Jewish values, there are few absolutes that outweigh all other concerns, in all contexts. More typically, we encounter dialectical tensions between competing moral interests that have specific contexts.

The Torah demands of us to act to save life. This crucial mitzvah is referred to as *piku'ah nefesh* (literally meaning "guarding a soul"). The biblical source for this mitzvah is the verse, "You shall not stand by while your fellow's blood is shed."[1]

But how far must we go? The Talmud explains:

From where do we know that if a person sees one's fellow Jew drowning, mauled by beasts, or attacked by robbers, that they are bound to save them? From the verse "You shall not stand by while your fellow's blood is shed." But is it derived from this verse? Is it not rather from elsewhere? Where do we know [that one must save one's fellow from]

---

1. Leviticus 19:16

the loss of themself? From the verse, "And you shall restore it [a lost object] to them!"[2] From that verse I might think that it is only a personal obligation, but that he is not obligated to take the trouble of hiring others [if one cannot save them oneself]; therefore, this verse teaches that one must [go to the extent of hiring others to save a life].[3]

Maimonides writes:

> If one person is able to save another and does not save them, they transgress the prohibition "You shall not stand by while your fellow's blood is shed." Similarly, if one person sees another drowning in the sea or being attacked by bandits, or being attacked by wild animals, and although able to rescue them either alone or by hiring others, does not rescue them; or if one hears a non-Jew or informers plotting evil against another or laying a trap for them and they do not call it to the other's attention and let them know; or if one knows that a non-Jew or a violent person is going to attack another and although able to appease him on behalf of the other and make him change his mind, they do not do so; or if one acts in any similar way – they transgress the prohibition "You shall not stand by while your fellow's blood is shed."
>
> Although one is not flogged for transgressing these prohibitions, because one only violates them through inaction,[4] the offense is most serious, for if one destroys [a] single life from Israel, it is regarded as though one destroyed

---

2. Deuteronomy 22:2
3. Babylonian Talmud, Sanhedrin 73a
4. The biblical punishment of lashes, or flogging, is only meted out when one transgresses by being active, and not by being passive as in the case of not saving a life.

the whole world, and if one saves a single life from Israel, it is regarded as though one saved an entire world.[5]

Should we, or must we, or *can* we, risk our own life to save another? The Hagahot Maimoniyot[6] writes:

In the Yerushalmi[7] it concludes that one is obligated to even enter into uncertain life-threatening danger [in order to save another from certain life-threatening danger].[8]

The Radbaz[9] takes this idea further:

…and not only this but even if there is a small amount of life-threatening danger [to the rescuer] like when one sees another drowning in the sea or being attacked by bandits, or being attacked by wild animals, in all of the cases there is some danger [to the rescuer]; even here one is obligated to save…One should know that included in the prohibition of "you shall not stand by," is that one [is] obligated to save another's property. However, one is not obligated to enter into uncertain life-threatening danger in order to save another's property. One *is* obligated to enter into uncertain life-threatening danger in order to save another's life or to prevent them from being sexually violated, and so it says it in the Yerushalmi. However, if the uncertainty of the danger inclines toward certain life-threatening danger, one is not obligated to give oneself over in order save another in danger.[10]

---

5. Mishneh Torah, Laws of the Murderer and Preserving Life 1:14–15
6. Rabbi Meir ben Yekutiel HaKohen of Rothenburg, Germany, 1215–1293
7. Jerusalem Talmud
8. Mishneh Torah, Laws of the Murderer and Preserving Life 1:14
9. Rabbi David ben Shlomo ibn Zimra, Egypt, 1479–1573.
10. Responsa, Radbaz 5:218

The Radbaz continues:

> It was asked of me to give my opinion on that which was written that if a non-Jewish ruler says to a Jew, "Let me cut off one [of] your limbs, that you will not die from, or I will kill your fellow Jew, [must he allow the authorities to cut off his limb?]" There are [indeed] those that say that one is obligated to let them cut off the limb, since one will not die…
>
> Answer: This is [only to be considered] acting righteously [beyond the letter of the law], but according to the letter of the law there is an answer…for perhaps through the cutting off of the non-essential limb, one will lose a lot of blood and die. Who is to say that the blood of your fellow is redder than your blood?[11] … Also, it is written: "Its paths are paths of pleasantness"[12] and it is essential that the laws of our Torah should agree with one's logic and common sense. Therefore, I see no reason for this ruling other than acting righteously [beyond the letter of the law]. Happy is the portion for one who is able to fulfill this. If there is uncertain life-threatening danger, one who risks one's life is to be considered a righteous fool, because [even] your uncertain danger takes precedence over your fellow's certain danger.[13]

Rabbi Herschel Schachter[14] writes:

> It happened in Brisk [Brestletovsk, Russia] that there was a cholera outbreak. Despite that it is a very contagious disease,

---

11. This is a Talmudic principle which means that your fellow's life does not take precedence over yours.
12. Proverbs 3:17
13. Radbaz 3:627
14. Contemporary Torah scholar and *halachic* decisor, New York.

Rabbi Chayim Soloveitchik[15] instructed that everyone in the town was obligated to help those that had passed out in the streets due to the illness and to help them in any way possible. Those that had passed out were to be considered to be in certain life-threatening danger while those who came to help them were only to be considered as if they are entering into uncertain life-threatening danger. Rabbi Chayim felt that the halacha is like Hagahot Maimoniyot in the name of the Yerushalmi[16] ... One time he even removed his own coat, even though by doing so he would endanger himself slightly by weakening his body from the cold and risk contracting cholera, in order to cover up one of the dangerously ill until they could be brought inside. The genius Rabbi Chayim did not become sick through this but many others who helped the sick did become sick and even die.[17]

Maimonides offers guidance on what to do about mitzvot that entail a small chance of injury:

It is important to know that the Torah does not take into account exceptional circumstances. But whatever the Torah teaches, whether it be intellectual, moral, or of a practical character, it follows the rule [of] the majority (of cases), and not that which is the exception ... It is not concerned with the injury that might be caused through a certain mitzvah or custom. For the Torah is Divine and (in order to understand its operation) we must consider how in nature

---

15. Rabbi Chayim Soloveitchik (1853–1918), also known as Reb Chayim Brisker, was a great Talmudic scholar and is credited as the founder of the popular Brisker approach to Talmudic study.
16. Notice that Rabbi Chayim Soloveitchik disagreed with the Radbaz on this point.
17. Nefesh HaRav, Rabbi Herschel Schachter, 166–167.

the various forces produce benefits that are general but, in a few cases, may also cause injury. This is clear from what we and others have said.[18]

Jewish law is also sensitive to suffering and when people should be allowed to die. We don't actively kill terminally ill patients; God forbid. But we can, under certain circumstances, stop engaging in interventions that keep them alive. Rabbi Moshe Feinstein[19] taught that one need not renew their oxygen tank when it runs out of oxygen for a dying patient who is suffering and does not have a chance of recovery. He ruled that this can also be applied to dialysis patients dying from renal failure who choose to not restart dialysis again.

We need to take pain and suffering seriously. The Magen Avraham[20] refers to a Talmudic story which recounts that when Rabbi Shimon bar Yohai and his son Eliezer were in hiding from the Roman authorities, they did not reveal their location to even Rabbi Shimon's wife (Rabbi Eliezer's mother). Magen Avraham writes:

> In Tractate Shabbat 33b (regarding the story of Rabbi Shimon Bar Yohai and the cave) it says that women are sensitive and if they are tortured, they might reveal the location [of Rabbi Shimon Bar Yohai and his son]. They then decided to go hide in a cave. From this we learn that it is permitted to flee from life threatening danger even though doing so will cause pain to your fellow. It also teaches that

---

18. *Guide for the Perplexed*, 3:34

19. 20th century, Russia and America. Rabbi Moses Feinstein was recognized as one of the greatest Torah scholars of the 20th century. He was unique in that even the highest regarded Israeli rabbis would defer to his decisions.

20. *Magen Avraham* was authored by Rabbi Avraham Abele Gombiner, 18th century Gabin (Gombin), Poland.

one is obligated to endure pain in order that one's fellow will not be killed.[21]

Rabbi Yaakov Emden[22] writes:

Also, it appears that one does not need to endure difficult suffering and bitterness in order to save their fellow because lashes are worse than death...All the more so one is not obligated to give [themselves] over to non-Jews to endure suffering in order to save their fellow.[23]

Should we, or can we, compel others by force to fulfill a mitzvah? On this question, Maimonides writes:

One who the law requires that he divorce his wife and does not want to do so, the rabbinic court in every place and time shall hit him until he says, "I want to [divorce her]." And the *get* [writ of divorce] will be written and it will be kosher [valid]. So too if Gentiles hit him and they say, "Do what the Jews say to you" and they pressure him until he divorces her – this is kosher...

Why does this not invalidate the *get*? Isn't this considered to be a case of a *get* forced against his will? Whether it was compelled by Jews or Gentiles, it is only considered to be "forced" when one is compelled to perform something that is not a mitzvah from the Torah, like buying or selling property. But one whose evil inclination has directed him not to perform a mitzvah or to do a sin, and physical force is used to get him to do that which he is obligated to or to distance him from something he shouldn't do, this is not considered "forced;" rather, [it is as if] he had previously been forced by his evil inclination.

---

21. *Magen Avraham*, Orah Hayim 156:2
22. 18th century Germany
23. Migdal Oz, Even Bochen 1:83

Therefore, one who does not wish to divorce his wife, since he wants to be a Jew, he [inherently] wants to do mitzvot and stay away from sin, and it is his evil inclination that has overtaken him, and since he has been beaten until his evil inclination became weakened and he said, "I want to...," he has divorced her according to his free will.[24]

So, indeed, according to Maimonides, one may, at times, be compelled to do what is right since ultimately, we can assume, everyone on the deepest level truly wants to do what is good and right. But if one does save another by their own altruism or by other motives, what does the rescued person owe to the rescuer? The Rosh[25] writes:

The one who is saved is obligated to compensate the rescuer for the expenses that the rescuer incurred. This is because one is not obligated to save another with one's own money if the one in danger has money. This is as was said in Tractate Sanhedrin 74a, "If one is being pursued and one's life is in danger, one is not liable for destroying the property of the pursuer in order to save one's own life. If one destroys the property of another to save one's own life, one is liable for the damage."[26]

Rabbi Yehoshua Falk haKohen Katz[27] writes:

It is [deduced] that one is obligated to save another in danger through their own efforts from the verse, "And thou

---

24. Mishneh Torah, Laws of Divorce, Chapter 2:20
25. Rabbi Asher ben Yehiel, late 13th, early 14th century Germany (later Spain after fleeing persecution)
26. Babylonian Talmud, Sanhedrin 8:2
27. (Poland 1555–1614). Rabbi Katz is better known by the title of his reputed work, the *Meirat Einayim*.

shall restore it to him."[28] From the verse, "You shall not stand by while your fellow's blood is shed,"[29] we [infer] the additional obligation that one must even spend money to hire another to save the one in danger if necessary. The Rosh and the Tur wrote that if the one in danger has money, they must compensate the rescuer. The Rosh brings a proof for this, and it is surprising that the Shulchan Aruch (and the Rema) did not cite this.[30]

Based on the biblical commandment to guard our own lives very carefully,[31] Rabbi Zvi Elimelech of Dinov teaches that the word מאד me'od (very) contains the same letters as the word אדם adam (human). He understands this to mean that the requirement to preserve health applies not just to one's personal health, but to the health of the human species. We must go to extremes to further health, for the only time the Torah uses me'od in a halachic context is here. We are obligated, beyond measure, to preserve our health and the health of others.

Only in the modern period have rabbinic decisors dealt with our exact question of whether it is permissible to be a living kidney donor. Some have ruled against it, basing their ruling on the opinion of Radbaz that we cited earlier: One who enters danger to save another person's life is hassid shoteh (pious fool).[32] Rabbi Yitzchak Weisz[33] argued in the early 1960s that the risk was too high,[34] and thus it was forbidden to donate

---

28. Deuteronomy 22:2
29. Leviticus 19:16
30. *Meirat Einayim*, Hoshen Mishpat 426:1
31. Deuteronomy 4:15
32. Radbaz 3:625
33. 1902–1989, Israel. Rabbi Weisz is better known by the name of his responsa, Teshuvot Minhat Yitzchak.
34. Teshuvot Minhat Yitzchak, 16:103. It is not possible to know how Rabbi Weisz and others of that era would rule today, as the procedure

one's kidney. Rav Eliezer Waldenberg[35] later agreed, until and unless the medical team says there is not a risk to donate.[36]

Rabbi Ovadia Yosef[37] also deals with the permissibility of donating a kidney.[38] Like others cited above, he sees this as a question of putting oneself in danger to save another. He explains further that the donor enters a *safeik sakanah* (possible danger) rather than a *vadai sakanah* (certain danger). He cites the Beit Yosef of Rabbi Yosef Karo who quotes the Jerusalem Talmud[39] and argues that not only is one allowed to put oneself in such a possible danger, one is obligated to do so. The Havot Yair[40] argues in favor of this obligation based on the famous Talmudic passage of sharing the flask in the desert:

> Two travelers in the desert have a canteen with water containing enough for [only] one to survive and reach a city. If they share the water, they will both die. Ben Peturah says, "Let them share the water, so that neither should see the death of his fellow." Rabbi Akiva says, "Let [one of them] drink the water, as it says, regarding the commandments, 'You shall live by them,' and not that you should die by them."[41]

---

is now considered much safer, and is more commonplace, than it was at that time.

35. 1915–2006, Jerusalem. Rabbi Waldenberg was highly sought after for his opinions on medicine and medical ethics.

36. Teshuvot Tzitz Eliezer 9:45

37. 1920–2013, Jerusalem. Rabbi Yosef was the Sefaradi Chief Rabbi of Israel, 1973–1983.

38. Teshuvot Yehaveh Da'at 3:84

39. Beit Yosef, Hoshen Mishpat 426. Also, see his Kesef Mishneh (commentary to Rambam's Mishneh Torah), Laws of the Murderer 1:14.

40. Havot Yair 126, authored by Rabbi Yair Bacharach, Germany 1639–1702.

41. Babylonian Talmud, Bava Metzia 62a

Rabbi Akiva rules that, in a case of certain danger, one traveler needs to drink the flask since both travelers are already in certain danger, and the traveler who drinks will likely survive. However, if sharing the water would put the traveler at only a possible risk, and would likely save the life of the fellow traveler, it would be a different situation with a different answer. Perhaps one may, or must, share the water as long as both travelers may survive.

Rabbi Ovadia Yosef argues, as we saw above, that it is indeed a mitzvah to donate one's kidney as a living donor. He adds that this is all the more so since the *safeik sakanah* (the possible risk) is a low risk. "It is certainly a mitzvah to donate [a kidney] to save one's fellow from certain death." Rabbi Ovadia later reiterates his earlier position,[42] and still later his son Rabbi Yitzchak Yosef [43] says that being a living kidney donor is a *"mitzvah rabbah"* (great mitzvah).

Rabbi Jonathan Sacks writes:

> There are two kinds of organ donations that do not pose problems in Jewish law. There are organ – a kidney for example – that can be taken from a living donor, who is taking little risk and remains healthy. Currently, 53 percent of all donors come under this category. We commend such donations and would encourage them wherever possible. At the other extreme, there are organs that can be taken when the heart of the donor has ceased to function, for example corneas and, again, kidneys. Currently 35 percent of kidney transplants fall into this category. Here, too, Judaism commends such donations.[44]

---

42. Teshuvot Yabia Omer 9, Hoshen Mishpat 12

43. Yalkut Yosef Hoshen Mishpat 426:6. Rabbi Yitzchak Yosef is the current Sefaradi Chief Rabbi of Israel.

44. Organ donation in Jewish law, *The JC*, January 2011, https://www .thejc.com/comment/opinion/organ-donation-in-jewish-law-1.20656

In sum, contemporary rabbinic sources widely regard donating organs (while living or after one's life) as a mitzvah – considered a commendable deed by some and an imperative by others.

Is one truly saving a life with a kidney donation? The Beth Israel Deaconess Medical Center in Boston explains:

> Patients who receive a kidney transplant typically live longer than those who stay on dialysis. A living donor kidney functions, on average, 12 to 20 years, and a deceased donor kidney 8 to 12 years. Patients who receive a kidney transplant before dialysis live an average of 10 to 15 years longer than if they stayed on dialysis. Younger adults benefit the most from a kidney transplant, but even adults as old as 75 gain an average of four more years after a transplant than if they had stayed on dialysis.[45]

The data is clear on what we're capable of achieving with a kidney donation. When a patient suffers from kidney disease, dialysis can keep the patient alive, but a kidney from a cadaver increases the recipient's life expectancy. A kidney from a living donor increases the life expectancy of the recipient significantly more, as highlighted in an article in *Nephro-Urology Monthly*:

> Although there were no significant differences in one-year survival rates of patient and graft between study groups, three-year survival rates of patient and graft were significantly longer in living donor kidney transplants than deceased donor kidney recipients.

Imagine a world where no one would die needlessly. For some diseases, we simply do not know how to save or prolong

---

45. "The Benefits of Kidney Transplant versus Dialysis," Beth Israel Deaconess Medical Center, https://www.bidmc.org/centers-and -departments/transplant-institute/kidney-transplant

life; but for kidney disease, we can indeed preserve and even prolong life. It is not easy or cheap, but is possible to prevent needless death.

Donating One's Body to Science

It is not difficult to make a *halachic* case for why one should not donate one's body to science. There are three primary concerns:

- The prohibition against leaving the body exposed[46]
- The prohibition against disrespecting the body[47]
- The prohibition against deriving benefit from a corpse[48]

Nonetheless, Rabbi Yitzhak HaLevi Herzog[49] offered a courageous *halachic* position in 1947, which is not well known, permitting donating one's body to science, because, albeit indirectly, the donation could potentially help to save a life. He writes:

> Do not object to the use of bodies of persons who gave their consent in writing, of their own free will during their lifetime, for anatomical dissections as required for medical studies, provided the dissected parts are carefully preserved so as to be eventually buried with due respect according to Jewish Law.[50]

Other *halachic* decisors overwhelmingly discouraged following Rabbi Herzog's ruling, although a significant few, Rabbi

---

46. Deuteronomy 21:23
47. Shulchan Aruch, Yoreh Deah 363, YD 367–368
48. Rambam, Laws of Mourning, 14:21
49. 1888–1959. He served as the first Chief Rabbi of Ireland, and later as the second Ashkenazi Chief Rabbi of Israel.
50. Myron Kolatch, "The Yeshiva and the Medical School" in *Commentary*, American Jewish Committee, Vol. 29, no. 5 (May 1960).

Eliezer Waldenberg (in the above quoted Tzitz Eliezer) and Rabbi Tzvi Pesach Frank[51] among them, concurred. While we have seen many sources in favor of organ donation for transplants; on the other hand, donating one's body for an autopsy, anatomy classes, or scientific research is highly discouraged in some Orthodox circles.

Even so, recently, Rabbi Dr. Yitz Greenberg and Rabbi Dr. Zev Farber have written an article arguing for the *halachic* permissibility of donating one's body to science with the aim of saving lives.[52] Their position is based on the view of Rabbi Yosef Messas[53] who also ruled that this is permissible, and even admirable. We cannot, according to Rabbi Messas, prioritize the bodies of the dead over the lives of the living.

---

51. 1873–1960. Rabbi Frank served as the Chief Rabbi of Jerusalem for several decades.
52. https://www.academia.edu/33749305/Autopsies_I_A_Survey_of _the_Debate?fbclid=IwAR32MLnexf5JVU8ROthc20c2OuZ0XO1e23 3mj90v__8UdktzMZ4CA-iNwSE
53. 1892–1974. Rabbi Messas served as the Chief Rabbi of Tlemcin, Algeria, later as the Chief Dayan (judge) of Meknes, Morocco, and later still as the Sefaradi Chief Rabbi of Haifa, Israel.

Chapter 3
Jewish Ethics

On Loving Strangers, Friendship, and Altruistic Relationships

Are human beings inherently selfish? Does something about human evolution force us – consciously or not – to look after only ourselves and those closest to us? There's no shame in looking after one's best interest. In fact, the Mishnah instructs us: "If I am not for myself, who will be for me?"[1] After all, if we don't advocate for ourselves, then the world around us could swallow us. Yet we admire people who at the same time look beyond their own immediate needs. We do not necessarily expect to find altruism in the rest of the animal kingdom.

Humanity, apparently, has the special ability to look out into the world beyond local and selfish desires – and seek greater purpose in serving others. Maybe we need that ability. Dostoyevsky wrote in *The Brothers Karamazov* that "Hell...is the suffering of being unable to love."

Feeling concern and love for someone we don't know should not be a burden. It is not heroic, but constitutive of our existential nature. Feeling compassion for those we don't

---

1. Pirkei Avot (Ethics of the Fathers) 1:14

yet love is a gift that expands us and enriches us. Compassion grants our world the merit to continue to exist. Each stranger we pass in the street has the potential to partner with us, to redeem us, and to be redeemed through us. Each individual can be a part of our spiritual story, if we so choose. We are all one family, members of an interconnected human race with a shared destiny. We deeply need one another.

When we ask to be happier, what we may really be asking for is the capacity to become more giving and loving. We are praying for an evolved heart that can contain more. We are capable of more than self-absorption. We do not want to become an individual as described by David Hume:[2] "...an individual cares more about the stubbing of his toe than a death on the other side of the world." Hume's individual prioritizes their own pain, and so feels sorry for himself. We want to expand our purview to include joy, both our own and of others. In the words of the Psalmist: "Teach me to feel joy as deeply as I feel sorrow."[3]

When we choose to give a kidney to save a stranger, we are not merely making a "sacrifice." We are not "losing an organ." Rather, we are gaining a soulmate – a family member. We gain a new dimension, a new perspective on existence, in which we can redeem the stranger and in turn become redeemed by the stranger. This is one of the radical teachings of the Torah – the Torah that is obsessed with our love and care for strangers.

We normally translate the famous Mishnaic dictum, "Who is rich? One who is content with his portion,"[4] as referring to what they themselves have. But another interpretation of the same phrase can be read as: "Who is rich? One who is content

---

2. 18th century British philosopher
3. Psalms 90:15
4. Pirkei Avot 4:1

with *another's* portion." When we feel that another's gain is in fact our gain, rather than feeling jealous, we feel joy at their success. Adopting this conception of wealth would constitute a real revolution, making our lives truly wealthy.

Humanity has the burden of understanding vast emptiness. We sometimes feel alone in the universe, as if we know no others in the expansive reaches of space. We must try to translate that feeling into caring for others who, no doubt, on occasion feel the same.

In the Torah, Joseph's father sends him to Shechem to look after his brothers, with whom he (Joseph) has a poisonous relationship. Joseph searches there and does not find them:

> And a man found him, when he was wandering in the field, and the man asked him, "What are you seeking?" And he said, "I am seeking my brothers" (Genesis 37:15).

For me, the story of Joseph has always resonated. As a child whose family moved to different cities regularly, I constantly felt like I needed "my brothers" to tell me that everything would be alright. As I've grown up, though, I've come to realize that to some degree, we all wander in search of our "brothers." We cultivate friendships with difficulty, made even more difficult for those of us who change locales often. We are increasingly *interdependent*, while our culture strangely latches onto the illusion of bold independence. In addition to friends who assist our journey, we seek life partners. At times we experience loneliness as a lamentable plague. At times we yearn to walk with others. Sometimes we succeed in finding friendship and love. When our relationships cultivate virtue, which I call "spiritual friendships," we remain grounded.

While friendship has a crucial role in child development, it does not lose its significance in adulthood, when we have the greatest opportunity to achieve virtuous living. The Talmudic rabbis strongly advise us to "acquire for yourself a friend."[5] Maimonides explains that "a person requires friends all their lifetime."[6] And like any other moral effort, this does not come naturally, but requires deliberation and toil.

Transience is not the biggest barrier to the cultivation of relationships today. Our obsession with the internet has undoubtedly weakened relationships. Fast-paced, self-interested connections on social media may tend to be less meaningful and more transactional. One can *friend* or *unfriend* someone with a simple click. While we collect many "friends" through social networking, these social bonds are often weak or vague at best. And while web-based friendships may initially be interesting, entertaining, and may even enhance our social capital in the short term, these digital links rarely create strong bonds in the long term. But we need strong bonds to foster morally-inspired living. We need friendship that involves less taking and more giving.

Today, we witness increased individualism, decreased institutional affiliation, and more talk about social networks than about relationships. Growing micro-communities may diminish our traditional communities. *True* friendship – where people can rely on each other through good times and bad – is on the decline. Nearly ten years ago, Cornell University sociologists found that adults typically have only two friends they can discuss "important matters" with – down from three in 1985. Half of those surveyed said they had only one; four percent had none.[7] Friendships may still be social and pleasant, but they are generally less confidential and intimate.

---

5. Pirkei Avot 1:6
6. *Guide for the Perplexed*, 3:49
7. Potter, More Facebook Friends, Fewer Real Ones, Says Cornell Study

In a friend, we find not only comfort and companionship but also moral accountability. The Scottish moral philosopher Alasdair MacIntyre, who frequently references Aristotle and other classical philosophers, explains: "In achieving accountability we will have learned not only how to speak to, but also how to speak for, the other. We will, in the home or in the workplace or in other shared activity, have become – in one sense of that word – friends."[8]

I do not suggest that the propensity to use social media has killed meaningful relationships, nor that we have lost the ability to cultivate virtue. Rather, I believe that religious communities have the opportunity to create consequential spaces for conversation, sharing, volunteering, and for creating mission-driven partnerships. Religious leaders and educators can help create micro-communities for students to discover friendship in the deepest sense, friendship that cultivates moral commitment and responsibility. This may be our most important role. Professors, social workers, and college counselors can help, but campus clergy are in the best position to create meaningful spaces for reflection, conversation, and service where students can cultivate deeply meaningful relationships.

The word for friendship in Aramaic is *havruta*, and this term connotes more than simply relationship. Rather, the term, among other things, encompasses the primary model of Jewish learning. A *havruta*, in its truest sense of the word, is a *bar plugta* – a challenger – one who not only supports us, but also challenges us. The Talmudic sage Rabbi Hanina teaches that in religious learning and growth, a friend is even

---

(ABC News November 8, 2011), https://d3jc3ahdjad7x7.cloudfront.net/zaLc3iJJvhACpwnvHQlx2DEe9MKlGqOZtLs2TDIifXEYbNlz.pdf.
8. See Alasdair C. MacIntyre, *Dependent Rational Animals: Why Human Beings Need the Virtues*, Open Court Publishing, Chicago, 1999.

more important than a teacher: "I have learned much from my teachers, but from my friends more than my teachers."[9] A friend of virtue can be connected to our intimate life pursuits more than any teacher can be. Thus, the rabbis teach that "one is not even to part from one's friend without exchanging words of Torah."[10] A friend, on this highest level, is primarily a learning partner, but also a supporting partner in forging a productive, well-rounded life.

While there is something to be said for socialization that comes naturally, we should not underestimate the role spiritual leaders can play to bring about friendships. Too often, religious leaders focus on building community to the exclusion of creating individual friendships. I've found that friendship on college campuses – probably among the most productive places for people to forge long-term relationships – is cultivated most deeply in spaces created solely for personal life reflection, openness, boundary-breaking, and trust-building activities.

Indeed, we engage in the deepest learning when in communication with an intimate companion. A relationship that involves mutual self-disclosure becomes no mere incident, but an opportunity for growth. In such a shared holy effort we cultivate solidarity and, in reciprocal transformation, we come to love one another; in such a relationship we co-construct our values, we discover our shared conception of *eudaimonia* (how best to live), and our identities become intertwined.

Jewish values motivate our commitment to supporting virtue-based friendship. To be sure, one clear and important value of friendship is utilitarian: friends help each other in times

---

9. Babylonian Talmud, Ta'anit 7a. The statement concludes, "and from my students most of all." The experience of teaching can also create moral partnerships.

10. Babylonian Talmud, Berachot 31a

of distress. The Book of Ecclesiastes expresses this utilitarian benefit of friendship: "Two are better than one, because they have a good reward for their labor. For if they fall, the one will lift up one's fellow; but woe to them that are alone when they fall, for they have not another to help them up."[11]

The Torah consistently reminds us to protect the stranger. In doing so, we can move the other, and ourselves, from alienation into a social network and friendship.

Rabbi Joseph B. Soloveitchik valued both a *"haver lede'agah,* a person in whom one can confide both in times of crisis, when distress strikes, and in times of glory, when one feels happy and content" and a *"haver lede'ah,* a person in whom he or she has absolute trust and faith."[12] A friend is an emotional partner on both our high and low journeys. Sometimes friendship is manifest in lifelong commitment. Other times, we can offer moments of the gift of friendship. People who are willing to connect to whomever they encounter are rarely socially – or existentially – lonely. Every moment can be seen as an opportunity for spiritual presence and friendship.

In addition to a support system, Rabbi Soloveitchik explains (based upon the Book of Job) that there is a vital spiritual purpose to friendships. "Job certainly did not grasp the meaning of friendship. At this phase, even communal and social relations served the purpose of utility and safety. Real friendship is possible only when a person rises to the height of an open existence, in which he is capable of prayer and communication. In such living, the personality fulfills itself."[13] It is not until Job

---

11. Ecclesiastes 4:9–10

12. Joseph B. Soloveitchik, *Family Redeemed,* Ktav, Jerusalem, 2000, 27–28.

13. Soloveitchik, *Out of the Whirlwind: Essays on Mourning, Suffering and the Human Condition,* Ktav Publishing House, Inc., Jersey City, NJ, 2003 ed., 64.

realizes the importance of opening himself spiritually to others that he truly comes to understand the virtue of friendship: "And the Lord returned the fortunes of Job when he prayed for his friends; and the Lord gave Job twice as much as he had before."[14]

Living a good, happy life without deep friendships was unfathomable to the Talmudic rabbis. According to one Talmudic story, Honi, the legendary miracle worker, outlived all his friends; he felt depressed when he experienced social isolation. He prayed for death so that he might be released from his despair. Rava[15] then uttered tersely that one must choose "either friendship or death."[16] We cannot thrive in our life without companionship.

When friendship morphs into a solely pleasure-seeking venture, it is less likely to be impactful or enduring; it is a momentary pursuit. But when friendship is about the cultivation of virtue, the opportunity to pursue the good, and the search for meaning, it can become enduring, even transformative. Friendships of pleasure and utility are fun but end as our needs and wants evolve. Friendships of virtue are not whimsical. Rather, they are attached to our pursuit of the just, holy, and good.

In a friendship infused with love, we yearn for unconditional love:

> Any love that is dependent upon a specific cause, when the cause is gone, the love is gone; but if it does not depend on a specific cause, it will never cease. What sort of love depended upon a specific cause? The love of Amnon for

---

14. Job 42:10
15. Rava is one of the most well-known Talmudic sages.
16. Babylonian Talmud, Ta'anit 23a

Tamar. And what did not depend on a specific cause? The love of David and Jonathan.[17]

Rabbi Samson R. Hirsch[18] writes about how we can actualize this love:

We are to assist in everything that furthers...well-being and happiness as if we were working for ourselves....For the demand of this love is something which lies quite outside the sphere of the personality of our neighbor...Nobody may look on the progress of another as a hindrance to his own progress, or look on the downfall of another as the means for his own rising, and nobody may rejoice in his own progress if it is at the expense of his neighbor...His own self-love too is only a consciousness of his duty. He sees in himself only a creation of G-d, entrusted to himself to attain the bodily, mental, and earthly existence, and for which He had given him directions in His Torah...He proclaimed his love of G-d, by his love to His creatures: *Oheiv et HaMakom, oheiv et Haberiyot* [a person who loves God loves people].[19]

In Jewish thought, love is not merely an emotion. Rather, love is made manifest through the deed. Rabbi Soloveitchik writes:

The Bible spoke of the commandment to love one's neighbor (Leviticus 19:18). However, in Talmudic literature, em-

---

17. Pirkei Avot 5:16. Note the difference in the language between "the love of Amnon *for* Tamar" and "the love of David *and* Jonathan."
18. 19th century, Germany. Rabbi Hirsch revitalized the Jewish community of Frankfurt and was a groundbreaking activist on behalf of Jewish education.
19. Commentary on Leviticus 19:18. For a related insight from one of the English Romantic writers, see Leigh Hunt's poem, "Abu Ben Adhem."

phasis was placed not only upon sentiment, but upon action, which is motivated by sentiment. The *Hoshen Mishpat*, the Jewish code of civil law, analyzes not human emotions but actual human relations. The problem of *Hoshen Mishpat* is not what one feels toward the other, but how he acts toward him.[20]

We emulate God when we act in a Godly manner in the world. We accomplish that elevated level of existence when we slide from a narrow consciousness in which we merely seek self-gain to an expansive consciousness where we seek for others to gain.

Kidney donation, especially altruistic donation which I hope will become the norm, creates one of the most beautiful extensions of friendship that we can cultivate: deep friendship, beautiful friendship, friendship not based upon external factors, but based on a gift – both physical and metaphysical. It creates deep companionship without equal anywhere in the world.

Without deep friendships, without deep love, we lack adequate self-knowledge and awareness of our blind spots. This leads to arrogance, as we become less able to recognize our need for others. To acquire most of our worldly knowledge, we must rely upon what others have shared with us to supplement our own experience. We look to experts for technical knowledge and to friends for subjective knowledge. When we fail to cultivate friendships, we fail to cultivate ourselves. To friends, we have special duties that arise from our relationship. Selfishness is anathema to friendship.

To become virtuous citizens committed to moral and religious excellence, we can benefit from influential figures. Religious leaders, family members, writers, artists, musicians, and

---

20. Soloveitchik, *Family Redeemed*, Ktav, Jerusalem, 2000, 40.

thinkers can reinforce the values that strengthen social bonds. We need these influences now, when bonds are increasingly threatened. When we cultivate bonds with others, we are destined to become more than we currently are.

Chapter 4
Spirituality

The Torah on Kidneys

Kidneys, in the idiom of the Hebrew Bible, give counsel. Inner conviction that English speakers associate with the heart, in biblical Hebrew comes from the kidneys. The Psalmist says, "I shall bless God, who counsels me, and even at night my *kelayot* (kidneys) instruct me."[1] Some translators make the text more comfortable and relatable for English readers and render the verse as "my heart instructs me," but this is a non-literal translation.[2]

An ancient Midrashic text draws on that verse to explain how Abraham discovered his inner conviction when there was no one to teach him.

> Said Rabbi Shimon: His father did not teach him, his rabbi did not teach him,[3] so from where did he (Abraham) learn the Torah? Rather the holy blessed One appointed his two kidneys like two rabbis, and they poured out and taught

---

1. Psalms 16:7
2. In the singular form, the Hebrew word for kidney is *kilya*. The verse uses the possessive *kilyotai* ("my kidneys").
3. Meaning, of course, that Abraham had no rabbi.

him Torah and wisdom. That is what is written: "I shall bless God, who counsels me, and at night even my kidneys instruct me."[4]

The rabbis were thinking about kidneys as symbols of spiritual impulses:

Our Rabbis taught: Man has two kidneys, one of which prompts him to good, the other to evil; and it is natural to suppose that the good one is on his right side and the bad one on his left, as it is written,[5] "A wise man's understanding is at his right hand, but a fool's understanding is at his left."[6]

I remember feeling grateful after learning this Talmudic passage and hearing that the medical team was planning, as usual, to remove the left kidney. I can report, though, that the *yetzer hara* (evil inclination) was still alive after the surgery. I wonder what the rabbis meant.

An old English expression associates kidneys with one's temperament or nature. One might say of one's son, "I hope he will be of similar kidney to his mother."

In some passages, the rabbis invoke both organs: "The kidneys prompt, the heart discerns." In the *Selichot* liturgy,[7] we say "*bochein kelayot valeiv*" (God searches one's kidneys and heart). There is wisdom and truth there. In a radical passage in the Book of Psalms, we learn that God "acquired" our kidneys in our mothers' womb.[8] This is to say that our kidneys never

---

4. Bereishit Rabbah 61:1
5. Ecclesiastes 10:2
6. Babylonian Talmud, Berakhot 61a
7. *Selichos,* Artscroll, p. 498, based on Jeremiah 11:20. Selichot are special prayers recited for several days leading up to Rosh HaShana and Yom Kippur.
8. Psalms 139:13

belonged to us! Was God already planning to use one of our kidneys for someone else's body? Was God preparing a cure before an illness even existed?

We are taught that one is like a newborn after doing *teshuvah* (repenting), or after Yom Kippur, or after a wedding or conversion. This can also be true after a transplant. One is reborn after having made oneself a *korban* (an offering to God): One quite literally lies down on the table as a *korban*, offering the body to God.

I was born at Mount Sinai Hospital (in Toronto, Canada) and I donated my kidney at Mount Sinai Hospital (in NYC); the name of the hospital serves as a reminder of my own personal rebirth. At Mount Sinai, the Jewish people convert (are reborn).

Rabbi Noach Isaac Oelbaum[9] taught (based on an idea in Hatam Sofer[10]) that as holy as the *Beit HaMikdash* (Temple) was, the life of one person is much, much greater! One life has more holiness than the *Beit HaMikdash* itself! Rav Oelbaum derives from this that giving a kidney to another should give one a greater joy than if one had personally built the *Beit HaMikdash*.

After the donation, I started to notice references to the word *kelayot* in the Tanach (Hebrew Bible), and I know that I will never miss them again. Eichah (the Book of Lamentations) compares the downfall of Jerusalem and the destruction of the Temple to injury to the kidneys.[11] Mentions of the kidneys are no longer just symbolic to me, but also literal messages about how to view our bodies.

---

9. Rabbi Oelbaum is a contemporary New York scholar and prolific lecturer.

10. Rabbi Moses Sofer, 1762–1839, Pressberg (Bratislava). Sofer means scribe; his actual family name was Schreiber.

11. Eichah 3:13

Often, if one hears that someone only has one kidney, they assume that they are a kidney donor. But it's not necessarily true.

About one in 750 people is born with only one kidney. The medical term for this condition, which is more common in men than women, is renal agenesis. Usually, it's the left kidney that is missing. Because it is possible to be healthy with one kidney, some people don't find out they have one missing until it's discovered on an X-ray or sonogram. (In another condition called renal dysplasia, the second kidney is present but does not function properly.)[12]

Indeed, God works in mysterious ways. Who is created with two kidneys and who with one? And why were people gifted two kidneys if they only need one to live? It seems more and more clear, to me, that the second kidney is there to potentially save the life of another.

When God told Abraham to go forth from his father's home, He instructs him, "*Lech lecha*," ("go for yourself"). Rashi famously says that "*Lech lecha*" here is meant in the literal sense,[13] "Go *to* yourself." Since Abraham specialized in and exemplified the mitzvah of *hachnasat orchim* (welcoming guests), he first needed to leave home to become a stranger himself in order to realize how much he was really helping others as a host. Sometimes we have to put ourselves on the other side to realize how much we're helping. Through my experience, I realized how important it is to support the sick.

---

12. "What's It Like to Live with One Kidney?" *Davita Kidney Care*, https://www.davita.com/education/ckd-life/whats-it-like-to-live-with-one-kidney.

13. The prefix (the Hebrew letter lamed) of the word "*lecha*" connotes both "for" and "to."

Our Five Deaths

In the sixteenth century, French philosopher Michel de Montaigne wrote: "To begin depriving life of its greatest advantage over us, let us deprive death of its strangeness, let us frequent it, let us get used to it....A man who has learned how to die has unlearned how to be a slave."[14] Certainly, one of the most serious and necessary aspects of religious epistemology is the way religion compels human beings to confront the void of death. While the philosophical meaning of such a proposition shall forever remain mysterious, a tangible byproduct of not knowing our ultimate fate gives us more than enough impetus to improve our lives and the lives of others around the world.

As an understandable consequence of the unknowable providence of death, the inevitability of it provides myriad spiritual and moral opportunities for us to learn and reflect. To be sure, the fear of death is only natural, but this palpable anxiety can yield productive action. After we have evolved through the five states of grief model articulated by Elisabeth Kubler-Ross (the familiar cycle of denial, anger, bargaining, depression, and acceptance), we can begin to transcend prior emotional states to have our own deaths motivate and inspire our own humble actualizations.

Because of the psychological clichés about death that are so prevalent in society today, I would like to propose a newer, more radical metaphysical model – one that describes how each person dies at five distinct moments in temporal time:

1. When we stop loving life and living to our full potential
2. The irreversible cessation of our heartbeat (or the death of the brainstem)
3. When our body is lowered into the earth

---

14. Montaigne's Essays

4. The last time our influence has any direct impact through posterity
5. The last time our name is ever mentioned on Earth

With each death, there is a tendency to have an unnatural and unhealthy response:

1. When we stop loving life and living fully – we can **seek a vacuous shell of empty ecstasy** and pleasure.
2. With the fear of the irreversible cessation of our heartbeat – **we can obsess upon the external health of the body.**
3. With angst about the moment when our body is lowered into the earth – **we can seek materials over love.**
4. Knowing that our impact will fade – **we can seek unilateral control** over our legacy.
5. Embracing that we will be forgotten – **we can try to build an ostentatious reputation** rather than one of humility.

In the nineteenth century Rabbi Simcha Bunim of Przysucha, one of the great Hasidic teachers of the age, relayed his own concise epitaph. On his deathbed, with his wife crying hysterically, he turned toward her and urged silence: "My whole life was only that I should learn to die." Likewise, the rabbis taught that a baby enters the world with fists clenched and a person dies with palms open to signify that we enter wanting everything of this world but we leave modestly, taking nothing with us.[15]

Only two things will remain after all five of our deaths: our eternal soul and the indirect effects of all we put into the world. As we edge closer to the precipice of death, we must strive, carefully and wisely with all of our might, to cultivate our eternal soul and to put positivity into the world. That in the end is all that will last.

---

15. Ecclesiastes Rabba 5:14

Chapter 5
Medical Dimensions

Dialysis: An Overview

Modern medicine is akin to the miracles of old, defying the mind. And the finest minds the world has ever known used their acuity and creativity to study and think of ways to mitigate – and sometimes outright cure – diseases that have afflicted humanity for millennia. Yet, with all the progress through better techniques in epidemiology, diagnosis, and cure, many conditions still cause bodily destruction. One of these, kidney disease, sadly remains. We do not yet have the ability to create an internally replicated kidney.

For far too many, dialysis is the only link separating life from death. Life on dialysis is hard.

To live on dialysis – a process that mimics the natural filtering performed by healthy kidneys – is to live with inconvenience, discomfort, expense, and fear. It is not a pleasant way to live. Some people can live on dialysis for only a few years. Others can tolerate the treatment and survive as long as twenty or thirty years. The average is, sadly, only five to ten years.[1]

---

1. "Dialysis" *National Kidney Foundation*, https://www.kidney.org/atoz/content/dialysisinfo.

While medical researchers described theoretical models for dialysis as early as 1854,[2] and several pioneers attempted to implement the procedure in practice, the first practical application of a "dialyzer" for acute renal failure was built in 1940. The Dutch physician Willem Kolff[3] began his research on dialysis when the Nazis invaded the Netherlands in 1940. Faced with the need to care for many wounded Dutch soldiers, he stepped up his efforts to construct a dialysis machine. Working in secret with his wife and a few colleagues – he faced arrest if discovered – Dr. Kolff used a washing machine, old cans, and various other improvised items to construct a working dialysis system using cellophane membranes and a rotating drum. In 1945, he achieved the first successful treatment with a 67-year-old patient in uremic coma with acute renal failure, who regained consciousness after eleven hours of hemodialysis with Kolff's dialyzer.

When the war ended in 1945, Dr. Kolff donated his machines (he had created five working models) to hospitals around the world, and lectured on dialysis. His machines were used for the next decade (although Mt. Sinai Hospital in New York, one of the recipients, initially rejected his ideas). Each early dialysis session required an incision, which limited the procedure to treating acute renal failure. Eventually doctors developed a procedure to use in-place tubes rather than fresh incisions. Now those in chronic end–stage renal failure could benefit from dialysis, enabling many to stay alive while they wait for a transplant.

---

2. "Brief History of Hemodialysis" Advanced Renal Education Program. https://advancedrenaleducation.com/wparep/article/history-of-hemodialysis/.

3. "The History of Dialysis" *Davita Kidney Care,* https://www.davita.com/treatment-services/dialysis/the-history-of-dialysis.

Now, decades after Dr. Kolff's first efforts, dialysis is widely used to treat symptoms of renal failure.

There are two kinds of dialysis:

In hemodialysis, blood is pumped into an artificial kidney (known as a hemodialyzer)[4] to be filtered. This involves minor surgery to create an access point to the patient's blood supply. If the patient has adequate blood vessels, the access point can be in the arm, using either a fistula (a surgically joined artery and vein) or a graft. If the patient's veins cannot support this, the access point can be a catheter inserted into the neck. Catheters are usually used for temporary access but can be used long-term if necessary. A person on hemodialysis must take great care of the access site to prevent infection. Some people can undergo hemodialysis in-home, but this requires four to seven treatments a week as opposed to the typical three at a dialysis center.

In peritoneal dialysis, a catheter is inserted surgically into the peritoneal cavity (abdomen) and the area is filled with dialysate, a fluid that purifies the blood within the body. There are two forms of peritoneal dialysis: *Automated* peritoneal dialysis uses a machine to filter out the fluid in the peritoneal cavity. *Continuous ambulatory* peritoneal dialysis does not necessarily require the use of a machine, providing a more practical form of treatment. Instead, the patient drains the fluid in and out of their peritoneal cavity via a plastic bag connected to a tube in the abdomen. This way a person may go about their normal daily life while on dialysis. The patient must do the entire exchange (in and out of the peritoneal cavity) three to five times a day.

Individuals need dialysis, whether hemo- or peritoneal,

---

4. "Dialysis" *National Kidney Foundation,* https://www.kidney.org/atoz /content/dialysisinfo.

when they no longer have healthy kidneys that can perform their biological function; this is a sign of end–stage kidney failure, usually when the kidneys have lost 85–90% of their functionality. Through dialysis, waste, salt, and extra water that the kidneys can no longer excrete naturally are filtered, and the body can keep a safe balance of potassium and sodium while maintaining healthy blood pressure. A person with chronic or end–stage kidney failure does not get healthier or cured on dialysis; rather, the person is kept alive, often for a limited amount of time. In some cases, a doctor will allow a patient on dialysis to be added to a kidney transplant waiting list.

Approximately 110,000 people begin dialysis in the United States annually, with the annual mortality rate within this group at about 20%.[5] The current trend is to hold off beginning dialysis until later in treatment, while trying (especially for the elderly) more conservative means to maintain kidney function. Researchers look for increased use of peritoneal dialysis, so that kidney patients can get their treatment in more locations (including the home) and more economically.[6]

Hemo- and peritoneal dialysis have the same level of effectiveness. Even so, peritoneal dialysis remains underutilized because caregivers frequently do not tell patients about this at-home treatment option.[7] The current kidney failure treatment

5. Kam Kalantar-Zadeh, "The Future of Dialysis in the U.S." https://www.renalandurologynews.com/home/departments/commentary/the-future-of-dialysis-in-the-u-s/.

6. Ram Gokal, "Peritoneal Dialysis in the 21st Century: An Analysis of Current Problems and Future Developments," *Journal of the American Society of Nephrology* 13 (suppl. 1) (January 2002) S104-S115, https://jasn.asnjournals.org/content/13/suppl_1/S104.short.

7. Jake Harper, "Why A Cheaper, More Convenient Dialysis Option Isn't More Common," August 7, 2018, https://www.sideeffectspublicm

industry centers on hemodialysis, so doctors are less incentivized to administer peritoneal dialysis.

Those who study the sector of the American healthcare system that conducts dialysis have criticized it for its lack of innovation, although progress is constantly being made. The mortality rate for patients on dialysis is steadily decreasing, due to efforts to ensure better quality of care at treatment centers, and especially to a decrease in dialysis-related infections. A quality incentive program and rating system has improved overall care, and the Centers for Medicare and Medicaid Services launched the *Fistula First Catheter Last* program in 2003, encouraging healthcare providers to use a fistula rather than catheters. The fistula, a less invasive procedure, has a much lower infection rate. New medications to treat early stages of renal failure have slowed the progression to end–stage renal failure.[8]

Each year, roughly half a million people are on dialysis – a lifesaver, but with all the drawbacks mentioned above. Scientists and healthcare providers hope to do better in the future. Currently, scientists are developing mobile artificial kidneys, which mimic the functions of normal kidneys, and can be attached externally or implanted in the patient. A completely effective artificial kidney would eliminate the need for kidney donations, greatly increasing the survival rates for those in end–stage renal failure. Although this would be a beneficial development, the technology is still many long years away.

Our best alternative today to sustaining patients with dialysis is saving lives with kidney transplants. Not everyone can

edia.org/post/why-cheaper-more-convenient-dialysis-option-isn-t-mo re-common.

8. Mahesh Krishnan & Kent Thiry, "Innovation in Dialysis: Continuous Improvement and Implementation," Last modified February 27, 2019, https://catalyst.nejm.org/innovation-dialysis-continuous-improvement/.

(or is willing to) donate a kidney, but most of us can advocate for those who desperately need to escape the prison of renal failure. Most of us can encourage donations. We have the opportunity to lead the community in making transplants more available as alternatives to the dialysis clinic. We can build society on a more ethical foundation.

What Happens During a Kidney Transplant?

A kidney transplant is complicated – before, during, and after the procedure itself. The transplant should begin right after harvesting the kidney from the donor, to keep the kidney in the best possible condition.[9] The surgery is complex and usually takes about three hours.

An anesthesiologist puts the patient under general anesthesia and monitors the patient throughout the entire procedure.[10] The surgeon puts the kidney in a different location in the body than where kidneys normally rest, a procedure called heterotopic surgery. (Orthotopic surgery, used for other organ transplants, such as heart and liver, puts the organ in its usual place). Original kidneys rest in the upper dorsal (back) abdomen; surgeons put the transplanted kidney in the lower frontal abdomen, near the pelvis. Unless the old, damaged kidneys cause complications, surgeons usually just leave them in place. If the damaged kidneys cause uncontrollable high blood pressure, or have recurring infections, or have become too enlarged, the surgeon has to remove them.

Once the patient is under anesthesia, the surgeon makes an incision in the lower abdomen, where the new kidney will

---

9. "Kidney transplant: What happens," https://www.nhs.uk/conditions/kidney-transplant/what-happens/.

10. "Kidney Transplant," *UCSF Department of Surgery*, https://transplant.surgery.ucsf.edu/conditions--procedures/kidney-transplant.aspx.

be placed. This location, either on the right or left side of the body, allows for the new kidney to be easily connected to the bladder and nearby blood vessels.[11] The surgeon then attaches a vein and an artery from the pelvic area to a vein and artery of the transplanted kidney, to supply it with adequate blood flow. The surgeon attaches the ureter (the tube which carries urine) of the donated kidney to the patient's bladder. A stent, a small plastic tube which aids in effective urine flow, may be placed in the ureter during the procedure and removed six to twelve weeks after, giving the body time to adjust to the new kidney. Once everything is in place, the surgeon will close the incision with surgical skin staples or stitches. A catheter will then be placed through the urethra into the bladder to allow urine to drain while the internal stitches heal.

Risks in Kidney Donation

One of the most significant barriers to a wider public willingness to undergo live kidney donation – and organ donation in general – is the fear of irrevocable bodily risk; opening our bodies is a frightening prospect. No one should feel shame for feeling scared about the consequences of living organ donation. Thankfully, when we talk openly about the risks of kidney donation, we come to a greater understanding and can evaluate the procedure more realistically. The donor really needs to be mentally prepared. While live kidney donation is generally quite safe, the procedure still presents risks. Nephrectomy (surgically removing a kidney) comes with risks of hemorrhage and infection, as do all surgeries.[12]

---

11. "Kidney Transplant Procedure: Procedure Details," *Cleveland Clinic*, https://my.clevelandclinic.org/health/treatments/4350-kidney -transplant-procedure/procedure-details.
12. "Living Kidney Donation," *UC Davis Health Transplant Center*, https://

Patients should start to walk on the night after the surgery, to facilitate healing. They can usually leave the hospital just days after the surgery. The donor should not do heavy lifting for four weeks and should not return to work for four to six weeks (this period of convalescence is longer for one who has to do heavy lifting at work). While the recipient's health insurance usually covers the basic cost for the donor, the donor should have health insurance coverage as well, to provide long-term care and follow-up. The only long-term lifestyle change is for donors to avoid contact sports.

Most surprisingly and fortunately for those who choose to donate, a donor's remaining kidney enlarges over time to handle its increased need to filter waste from the blood.[13] This natural adjustment is important because the kidney is critical to maintaining healthy blood pressure. Healthy kidneys produce the hormone aldosterone,[14] which regulates blood pressure by increasing the amount of sodium reabsorbed into the bloodstream and by increasing the amount of potassium excreted.[15] High blood pressure would damage the kidneys, preventing proper filtering of waste and impeding the production of aldosterone, which would in turn progressively damage the kidneys.

health.ucdavis.edu/transplant/livingkidneydonation/living-kidney-donation.html.

13. "What to Expect After Donation," *National Kidney Foundation,* https://www.kidney.org/transplantation/livingdonors/what-expect-after-donation.

14. "How High Blood Pressure Can Lead to Kidney Damage or Failure" Heart.org, https://www.heart.org/en/health-topics/high-blood-pressure/health-threats-from-high-blood-pressure/how-high-blood-pressure-can-lead-to-kidney-damage-or-failure#.WZjhfq3MwxI.

15. "Aldosterone" *The Society for Endocrinology,* https://www.yourhormones.info/hormones/aldosterone/.

After donating a kidney, the one remaining kidney typically grows to take on all the function of two healthy kidneys.

Potential donors often worry about the impact of a nephrectomy on their general health and longevity. A 2013 study theorized (on the basis of computer simulation) that donor longevity would be reduced by nearly a year for 40-year-old white men, slightly more for white women, and more for black donors. The study projected results from indications that nephrectomy is associated with less efficient filtering of excess water (lower glomerular filtration of water), with filtering out proteins that should remain in the blood (called proteinuria), and with higher blood pressure.[16] However, this simulation has not been borne out by clinical data. In a 2010 article published in JAMA (the *Journal of the American Medical Association*), researchers compared health results of more than 80,000 live donors against healthy matched controls over a 15-year period (1994–2009). While the 90-day mortality was higher for live donors (25 of 80,347, or about 3 per 10,000 nephrectomies vs. 0.4 per 10,000 in the healthy cohort), "long-term mortality was similar or lower for live kidney donors than for the matched … cohort throughout the 12-year period of follow-up."[17]

Men, African-Americans, and Hispanics had higher than average rates of post-donation mortality; donors with hypertension had the highest 90-day mortality (more than nine times the average). In addition, the researchers in the 2010 clinical

16. Bryce A Kiberd, "Estimating the long-term impact of kidney donation on life expectancy and end stage renal disease," Transplantation Research, 2:2, 2013, https://www.ncbi.nlm.nih.gov/pmc/articles/PMC3577426/pdf/2047-1440-2-2.pdf.

17. Dorry L. Segev, Abimereki D. Muzaale, Brian S. Caffo, "Perioperative Mortality and Long-term Survival Following Live Kidney Donation." JAMA, 303(10):959–966, 2010, https://jamanetwork.com/journals/jama/fullarticle/185508.

study noted that donor mortality dropped significantly in more recent years (between 2006–2009), indicating a "learning curve" that they predicted would result in even lower future mortality. At present, most scientific estimates support the conclusion that nephrectomy in healthy donors does not reduce donor longevity and does not increase donor risk for kidney disease.[18]

Not everyone can be (or should be) a donor. Out of concern for the donor's health, people with certain health-related issues are usually not good candidates for kidney donations, although even they are not necessarily ruled out. These issues include hypertension, diabetes, conditions affecting major organs (kidney disease, cardiovascular disease, liver disease), and sickle cell disease, which make people more susceptible to renal failure and other complications. Out of concern for the recipient, people with hepatitis or human immunodeficiency virus (HIV) usually cannot donate, since these illnesses can be transmitted through transplant.

Someone considering donating a kidney should undergo rigorous health tests such as an electrocardiogram, a blood pressure check, kidney and liver function tests, heart and lung disease evaluation, and tests to determine whether the person had past viral illness or another preexisting contraindication. A computer tomography (CT) scan combined with X-rays will determine whether kidney function is normal. Equally essential, before undergoing the procedure, the potential donor should have a psychosocial evaluation to ensure that they are emotionally and socially ready for the nephrectomy. Only after all these tests can the potential donor be cleared for the

---

18. "Living Kidney Donation," *UC Davis Health Transplant Center*, https://health.ucdavis.edu/transplant/livingkidneydonation/living -kidney-donation.html.

nephrectomy. These measures are necessary to ensure the procedure is a success for everyone involved.

Even with these extensive measures, we need to watch out for new risks. For example, the current opioid epidemic may have an impact on donations. A recent study demonstrated that kidney donors who had used opioids within a year before their nephrectomies were significantly more likely to experience subsequent hospitalization than donors who had not.[19] As result, those who have used opioids in the past, whether recreationally or for medical reasons, may be discouraged from donating. All of these precautions are taken in order to ensure that a donor nephrectomy remains a safe procedure.

The cost of the nephrectomy can present a barrier and prevent people from following through on a plan to donate a kidney.[20] Although the recipient's insurance usually covers many parts of the process for the donor, some costs are not covered, including lost wages, transportation, and other ancillary costs. If the donor doesn't have insurance, the donation may cause undue financial stress. Even with insurance, some insurance companies don't cover organ donation, viewing it as an unnecessary operation; the donor would face no harm from forgoing the procedure, and the operation might even put the donor at increased risk. We need to remove financial barriers to donation to increase the rate of donation and save more lives.

19. KL Lentine et al. "Predonation Prescription Opioid Use: A Novel Risk Factor for Readmission After Living Kidney Donation," *Am J Transplant*, 17(3):744–753, March 2017, https://www.ncbi.nlm.nih.gov/pubmed/27589826.

20. "The Side Effects of Becoming a Living Kidney Donor," Kidney.org, https://www.kidney.org/blog/kidney-cars/side-effects-becoming-living-kidney-donor.

The Amazing Capacity of the Human Kidney

The human body, which we easily take for granted, is truly a marvel. Focus your attention on the beauty of its complexity, the multiple systems working in harmony in ways we cannot totally comprehend, and the body inspires awe. Indeed, it's amazing that an organ only the size of a fist can contain millions of small blood vessels capable of such intricate wonders, and can last a lifetime if we are wise enough to treat it well.[21] I'm referring to the kidneys, those crucial organs that filter waste from our blood while retaining useful substances such as protein and red blood cells. The kidney's filtering process excretes waste materials through urine. Incredibly, a kidney also produces hormones that support other organs, helps provide regulation of blood pressure, and controls the delicate fluid balance within the body.[22]

As a result of the kidney's many functions and constant interactions with waste, it can be extremely sensitive. Drugs that help us in some ways may damage our kidneys. Medications that can cause acute renal injury include analgesics[23] (painkillers), antibiotics, chemotherapy drugs, and some drugs used for hypertension.[24] Physicians use tests to check for chronic kidney disease. These involve testing for protein in the urine and

21. "Kidney Disease (Nephropathy)" *American Diabetes Association*, http://www.diabetes.org/living-with-diabetes/complications/kidney-disease-nephropathy.html.

22. Barry M. Popkin, Kristen E. D'Anci, & Irwin H. Rosenberg. "Water, Hydration and Health," *Nutrition Reviews vol. 68,8* (2010): 439–58. doi:10.1111/j.1753-4887.2010.00304.x.

23. "Pain Medicines (Analgesics)" *National Kidney Foundation*, https://www.kidney.org/atoz/content/painmeds_analgesics.

24. "What Meds Might Hurt My Kidneys?" *WebMD*, accessed July 2, 2019 from https://www.webmd.com/a-to-z-guides/medicine-hurt-kidneys#1.

for serum creatinine, a chemical waste product resulting from the metabolism of muscle.[25]

These tests are necessary, because in type 2 diabetes, the kidneys are overburdened due to high blood sugar (known as hyperglycemia), and waste backs up in the kidneys. When that happens, the kidneys can, instead of leaving protein in the blood, let protein leak into the urine. Damaged kidneys can fail to remove creatinine, a waste product, so doctors test for kidney function by measuring creatinine in blood (serum creatinine). The higher the number, the poorer your kidney function. Compare the results with normal values and track the results over time, and you can see if your kidney function is declining or healthy.

Nephrologists[26] can study and treat dozens of kinds of kidney disease. Some renal conditions require the removal of a kidney (nephrectomy). For other conditions, the kidney can stay in the body, but renal function is so poor that one needs to be on dialysis to ensure proper filtering of blood.[27] Thankfully, nephrologists can now treat kidney diseases that were once inevitable death sentences.

We can take proactive steps to keep our kidneys healthy: eating healthy diets, exercising, and drinking sufficient fluids all allow the kidneys to filter waste. These practices also help prevent high blood pressure, which can lead to renal damage or failure.[28] Type 2 diabetes is the leading cause of kidney disease, and many people with diabetes also have hypertension

---

25. "Creatinine blood test" *MedlinePlus,* U.S. National Library of Medicine, https://medlineplus.gov/ency/article/003475.htm.
26. Nephrologists are doctors specializing in issues related to the kidney.
27. "Kidney Failure," *Barnes Jewish Hospital,* https://www.barnesjewish.org/Medical-Services/Transplant/Kidney-Transplant/Kidney-Failure.
28. Popkin, D'Anci, & Rosenberg, "Water, Hydration and Health," *Nutrition Reviews vol. 68,8* (2010): 439–58. doi:10.1111/j.1753-4887.2010.00304.x.

(high blood pressure), another common cause of kidney disease. Other kidney diseases can strike without warning or without known cause. Polycystic kidney disease runs in families, tragically attacking one relative after another. Some people are born with congenital kidney abnormalities. Some people (men, typically), for example, absorb too much calcium and develop kidney stones that can be extremely painful or even life-threatening.

Several drugs can treat symptoms of diseases that often occur alongside renal failure, such as hypertension and diabetes.[29] Some of those drugs themselves can harm the kidneys, so care must be taken to follow any medically prescribed protocol exactly. On the other hand, blood pressure drugs called ACE inhibitors and ARBs apparently delay the loss of kidney function in some patients.[30] Lifestyle changes make important contributions to disease treatment. Every aspect of a person's lifestyle affects the kidneys. If you feel concerned about your kidneys, you should limit any interaction with recreational drugs and alcohol. During early stages of kidney disease, you can tolerate a small amount of alcohol, but the kidneys do have to work hard to filter it out. Alcohol should not be a regular part of your menu if you suffer from kidney disease.

In later stages of renal failure, patients might need to alter food and water consumption. People adopting a kidney-friendly diet have to decrease the amount of sodium, potassium, phosphorous, and even water they consume. Typically, they should cap sodium and potassium intake at 2,000 mg a day, and phos-

---

29. "Treatment – Chronic kidney disease," *National Health Service,* https://www.nhs.uk/conditions/kidney-disease/treatment/.

30. "Keeping Kidneys Safe: Smart Choices about Medicines," *National Institute of Diabetes and Digestive and Kidney Diseases,* https://www.niddk.nih.gov/health-information/kidney-disease/keeping-kidneys-safe.

phorus at 1,000 mg.[31] Some patients need to increase, and some to decrease, intake of proteins.[32] Excess water intake may make it harder for the kidneys to function properly, so patients may have to lower the amount of water they drink, at least before beginning dialysis treatments. Tragically, many kidney diseases are not yet fully understood.

In still later stages of renal failure, patients require dialysis or even transplantation, each of which fortunately has a high success rate.[33] Once a patient's kidney function is critically low, even if the patient has not started dialysis, doctors will offer the option of transplantation. If the patient knows someone willing to donate a kidney – preferably a relative with the same blood type, in order to lessen the risk of rejection – that will likely result in a timely transplant. If not, then the patient can wind up on a transplant list. The transplant list, although the fairest way of determining how kidneys are distributed, is complicated and can leave a patient waiting for years.[34] Despite how it sounds, the transplant list does not assign donations in first-come, first-served order. When an organ becomes available, a computer algorithm calculates who gets the organ, ranking recipients according to several factors, including compatibility.

---

31. Kaitlyn Berkheiser, "17 Foods to Avoid If You Have Bad Kidneys," https://www.healthline.com/nutrition/foods-to-avoid-with-kidney -disease#section1.

32. Ko GJ1, Obi Y, Tortorici AR, & Kalantar-Zadeh K, "Dietary protein intake and chronic kidney disease," *Curr Opin Clin Nutr Metab Care,* 20(1):77–85 (Jan 2017) https://www.ncbi.nlm.nih.gov/pubmed/27801685.

33. "Kidney Transplant" *National Institute of Diabetes and Digestive and Kidney Diseases,* https://www.niddk.nih.gov/health-information/kidney -disease/kidney-failure/kidney-transplant.

34. "How Organ Allocation Works," *U.S. Department of Health & Human Services,* https://optn.transplant.hrsa.gov/learn/about-transplantation /how-organ-allocation-works/

While on the transplant list, patients get monthly tests to ensure that the best kidney is given to the right recipient. When, and if, the patient becomes assigned to receive a kidney, he or she will need the surgery as soon as possible. Unfortunately, there is always risk of organ rejection, which occurs when the body does not recognize the kidney as its own, causing the immune system to attack it. Though we need our immune system to protect against infection, early heart disease, and other disorders,[35] a full-strength immune system potentially endangers transplants. Medications weaken or suppress the immune system to lessen the risk of rejection; it is a serious cost, but better than not getting the transplant at all.

Sometimes, unfortunately, our efforts at immunosuppression fail. The transplant triggers strong reactions from the immune system, called immune mediated kidney diseases, which endanger any future kidney donation.[36] Glomerulonephritis, the immune-mediated inflammation of the glomeruli (tiny filters in the kidneys), is responsible for approximately 18% of kidney transplant failures.[37] For people with these diseases, a transplant may temporarily prolong their lives, but they are likely to experience the disease in their new kidney as well.

Today, nephrologists look for methods to improve and simplify the process of immunosuppression. A promising future

---

35. Mohamed H Sayegh, "Looking into the crystal ball: kidney transplantation in 2025," *Nature Clinical Practice Nephrology* volume 5, page 117 (2009). https://doi.org/10.1038/ncpneph1042.

36. John D Imig and Michael J Ryan, "Immune and inflammatory role in renal disease." *Comprehensive Physiology* vol. 3,2: 957–76. (2013) doi:10.1002/cphy.c120028.

37. J. Sellares et al. "Understanding the Causes of Kidney Transplant Failure: The Dominant Role of Antibody-Mediated Rejection and Nonadherence," *American Journal of Transplantation*, 14 September 2011, doi: 10.1111/j.1600–6143.2011.03840.x.

strategy may be kidney regeneration, literally growing a new kidney from the patient's own stem cells, which would avoid the need for immunosuppression and counteract the shortage of suitable donor organs.[38] Thus far, advancements such as stem cell research are only experimental, as the complexity that makes the kidney such an amazing organ is also the chief obstacle to regeneration. For example, the laboratory-grown kidney would need to create a complete vascular structure with millions of capillaries and larger blood vessels suitable for linking that structure to its recipient. This remains a problem with no quick solution. Still, patients could be spared from dialysis if even one-tenth of a healthy kidney's filtration capacity can be restored, so any progress in this direction could produce dramatic improvements.

A functioning kidney gives us the amazing ability to experience life to its fullest. Oftentimes, we don't even consider that these little organs have the power to determine our comfort and enjoyment of life. Progress to eliminate kidney disease is coming at a slow pace, but still, progress is apparent. In kidney disease, as in all medicine, we see continuing remarkable breakthroughs in our understanding of our body's processes. Some technological advances improve surgical procedures. Other scientific findings refine how we understand and treat aspects of our bodily functions. The kidney is, of course, no exception, and new advances continue to emerge.

While we wait for better solutions to ease the horrible weight of kidney disease, we already have two options in place to help those with renal failure: becoming living organ donors or donors after our passing. Post-mortem donation presents

---

38. Shuichiro Yamanaka and Takashi Yokoo, "Current Bioengineering Methods for Whole Kidney Regeneration," *Stem Cells International*, volume 2015, Article ID 724047, http://dx.doi.org/10.1155/2015/724047.

limited opportunities to save lives even when it does work. For this reason, we witness the rare opportunity to save life through the unique contemporary process of living kidney donation. It is a scary proposition to be sure, but one that can affect millions of vulnerable, scared people in a positive way.

The Scandal of Throwing Kidneys Away

The number of people who need a kidney is disproportionate to the number of kidneys available for donation at any given time. This is a modern human rights crisis happening without much notice, and it is a shameful dereliction of our obligation to assist vulnerable people. Each day, about twelve people die while waiting for a kidney transplant.[39] Yet, despite the need for more kidneys to save the lives of people living with renal failure, more than 3,500 useable donated kidneys are discarded every year in America. This is a scandal of the highest order.

These kidneys get dumped because of how the United States handles organ donation. Within the country, several different transplant programs organize the use of donated kidneys. Some programs pick and choose the best available kidneys for transplant. They sometimes prefer not to attempt a transplant at all unless the donated kidney is of the highest quality.

Generally, hospitals prefer higher quality kidneys that begin working faster after transplantation in order to avoid extra costs.[40] The less time it takes for a donated kidney to "wake up," the lower the long-term costs are for administrators, and most

39. Jen Christensen, "U.S. Is Discarding Too Many Potential Donor Kidneys, Study Suggests." CNN. Cable News Network, August 27, 2019. https://www.cnn.com/2019/08/26/health/thousands-of-kidneys -thrown-away/index.html.

40. Adrianna Rodriguez, "US Discards Thousands of Donated Kidneys Each Year as Patients Die on Waitlist, Study Says." USA Today. Gannett Satellite Information Network, August 30, 2019. https://www.usatoday

importantly, for patients. Medicare and Medicaid also put pressure on transplant programs and hospitals to have lasting and successful transplants, so the more unsuccessful transplants each program attempts, the less credibility the program will have. As a result, all donated kidneys are thoroughly inspected, and a kidney marked for a recipient may get rejected even if it is the best available for that patient.

Of the more than 150,00 kidneys donated between the ten-year span of 2004–2014, 28,000 of them – about 17% – were discarded. Although some donated kidneys must be discarded for medical reasons, many more kidneys than necessary get thrown away in the United States. It is a healthcare catastrophe. Indeed, a panel of organ transplantation specialists reviewing decisions to discard kidneys found that a staggering 50% which were designated to be discarded were actually suitable for transplantation.[41]

The United Network for Organ Sharing (UNOS), a nonprofit that manages the national organ waiting list, developed a scale for evaluating the quality of a donor kidney known as the kidney donor profile index (KDPI). The higher the KDPI, the lower the quality of the kidney and vice versa. To check the quality of the kidneys, organ procurement centers – which match available kidneys and transplant centers – often perform biopsies on the kidneys to test their long-term viability. The longer a kidney stays outside of the body, the less viable the kidney becomes, so repeated biopsies only lead to rejected

.com/story/news/nation/2019/08/29/us-throws-away-3-500-donated-kidneys-per-year-study-says-heres-why/2139644001/.

41. "Report of National Kidney Foundation Consensus Conference to Decrease Kidney Discards." National Kidney Foundation, October 23, 2018. https://www.kidney.org/news/report-national-kidney-foundation-consensus-conference-to-decrease-kidney-discards.

kidneys. Experts have pointed out that these biopsies aren't really necessary to prove compatibility. Given that almost none of the people who die every year can provide viable kidneys, the current model of kidney donation does not supply nearly enough kidneys to meet the demand.

Not every country approaches organ donation the same way the United States does. France, for example, practices a method known as aggressive kidney acceptance. The French reason that any kidney transplant, regardless of whether it will last five years or twenty, leads to a much better quality of life for a patient than continued dialysis. The yearly mortality rate of people on dialysis is 20%, meaning most people on dialysis don't make it past five years. So France uses kidneys that would be discarded in America. In America, kidneys from patients with preexisting conditions, such as diabetes or hypertension, are discarded even though they are usually perfectly viable for transplantation.

There is a contradiction between maintaining a high success rate and doing what needs to be done now to save lives. According to Dr. John Fung (see our interview coming up next in this book), much of the problem comes from a bureaucracy that imposes an actuarial intrusion on what should be a patient-centered decision to allocate donated organs to those who need them: "It is ridiculous to expect a 95% one year graft survival rate for kidney transplants... The quandary that we have been put into: UNOS allocating organs to sickest patients first but on the other hand [the Scientific Registry of Transplant Recipients and Centers for Medicare and Medicaid] penalizing centers for poor outcomes when we [doctors] try to do what we were supposed to do in the first place and help those high risk, very sick patients."[42]

---

42. Email from Dr. John Fung, "Fwd: The US Is Throwing Away at Least 3,500 Donated Kidneys Every Year, Study Finds." August 27, 2019.

In the end, is there a solution for America to stop throwing away precious kidneys (and other organs), depriving those who need the transplants most desperately? If the government of the United States were to adopt France's approach, it could prolong the lives of thousands of Americans. This is possible, not a pipe dream. A study published by *JAMA* states that if the U.S. were to adopt this strategy, transplant centers would be able to use about 62% of the currently discarded kidneys, which would generate 132,000 years of life across all recipients.[43] It is incumbent upon us, therefore, to lobby decision makers in the government and related agencies to reform organ donation policy so that vital organs are not left to rot when they don't have to be wasted. It is sickening to realize how many organs get thrown away like spoiled lunch meat.

We must do better. We must lobby those who control the system of organ donations. We must not fear shaking up the status quo: Too many people die as we cling to the old ways of organ donation. Why not innovate in organ matching and implantation? The antiquated impediments to partnering willing (or deceased) donors with desperate recipients needs to end, and fast. Let us be part of the solution – to do the best for everyone suffering from organ failure – through direct civic engagement.

What To Do When a Family Member Needs a Kidney

One of the most emotionally wrenching experiences one can have is seeing a family member suffer. For many families, the thought of seeing a loved one live every day in crippling pain because of organ failure – renal failure, specifically – is a slow form of torture. No family deserves to confront this agony, the lingering ferocity that kidney failure inflicts on body and soul.

---

43. Rodriguez, "US Discards Thousands of Donated Kidneys Each Year..." See note 40.

Though renal disease can cause excruciating pain for families, families are not helpless. Family members can take steps to bring relief and support to their afflicted loved one.

The first step is to ensure your loved one is on a donor registry, to start the process of their search for a kidney. The primary reason to sign up for the registry is the database matching system. The National Kidney Registry is the leader in the field. The Registry is exactly as it sounds: a list that includes thousands of names of people in search of a kidney.[44] Having more people included in the Registry, including potential donors, exponentially increases the likelihood of matching donor to recipient.

This leads to the second step: family members will want to get tested to see if any of them are a good match for the person in need. Getting tested, of course, is not a commitment to donate. It is merely a check to see if one is eligible to donate to a particular person. You might think that because you are not a perfect match (based on blood type and other factors) you cannot help. This is not true. By starting a chain and creating "paired donations," one can donate to someone else's loved one who is a better match, and that other person can donate to yours.[45] Sometimes, this can just involve two couples; other times, it can involve dozens of couples. Every transplant center works with UNOS (United Network for Organ Sharing) to coordinate the master list of donors and recipients in their database.

The third step a family member can take is to ensure that as many people as possible know about the need. Undeniably, it's difficult for some to take their story public. Still, this action is crucial. You should create and distribute a picture of your family

---

44. National Kidney Registry, https://www.kidneyregistry.org/.
45. "Kidney paired donation," *United Network for Organ Sharing*, https://unos.org/transplant/kidney-paired-donation/.

member, with their blood type, some contact information, and a message of hope. You should email it to your contacts, use social media, and write publicly wherever/whenever possible. Those who aren't used to being public advocates may find this step challenging, which is normal. But this challenge, while understandable, is outweighed by such a life-and-death matter.

As a family member, you have the ability to become a donor advocate for the recipient even if they are uncomfortable or unable to advocate for themselves. The more people involved in telling the story the better, so an advocacy team is always a good idea. Talking to others about the situation increases awareness and raises the chances of finding a donor. Whether or not you are the sole donor advocate for a recipient, organizing social events and fundraisers will help bring awareness to the situation, and give you more opportunities to share your loved one's story.[46]

Many people who approach me wonder if they are too old to donate. In fact, age is not necessarily a factor for donating. You can donate in your 60s, 70s, or even 80s, as long as you are in good health.

Several elements are important to include when sharing the story of a person in need. In addition to medical information such as the individual's condition, transplant need, and blood type, publicity should also touch on some of the logistics of a donation and transplant. This can include things like the location of the transplant, contact information, and information regarding what your insurance will cover, as well as the extra expenses – travel, for example – the donor might incur. Most importantly, however, remember to talk about the

46. Risa Simon, "5 Ways to Inspire Living Kidney Donation," *National Kidney Foundation,* https://www.kidney.org/newsletter/5-ways-to-inspire-living-kidney-donation.

person not as a sufferer of a disease, but as a symbol of hope and redemption. Talk about the patient's future plans and goals – and everything the person wants to live for. At first it may feel uncomfortable, but all you're doing is telling a story, not explicitly asking for donations. If someone wishes to be your donor, they will offer it to you.

Based on my own experiences, I believe that it's best to advocate for living donation, because living donation is more successful than post-mortem donation. Kidneys suitable for post-mortem donations show up when they do, where they do. The patient has to be patient, and wait for the opportunity, which may or may not come in time. When the opportunity comes, the transplant team has to make the best match it can, and then transport the kidney from wherever it happens to be to the recipient. They have to preserve the kidney during this trip, to keep it functional as long as necessary.[47] A donation from a living donor has none of these disadvantages. You can begin to schedule a live kidney donation relatively quickly, as soon as the patient needs one and a donor comes forward, compared to waiting for an appropriate cadaveric kidney to become available. The transplant team can remove the kidney from the living donor in one room and take it to the recipient next door. Getting the surgery on a prompt schedule, which happens with live donation, shortens the time on dialysis, and increases the chances of success. Live kidneys generally match the recipient better, last longer, and have lower rejection rates.

The medical team conducts tests to determine donor and recipient compatibility. The first, blood-type matching, is important because people have antibodies against blood types that are not their own. Human blood comes in four types: A, B,

47. "Why Do Living Kidney Donor Transplants Offer Better Outcomes?" *University of Minnesota Health,* https://www.mhealth.org/blog/2017/july -2017/why-do-living-donor-kidney-transplants-offer-better-outcomes.

AB, or O. For example, an A-type red blood cell has A antigens – markers on the cell that tell the body it belongs there.[48] The blood serum, however, contains antibodies against B antigens; so if someone with B-type blood donated to someone with A-type blood, the immune system would "attack and destroy" all the B-type cells. Therefore, a person with A blood could not receive a kidney from someone with B or AB blood. They could, however, receive from a person with O-type blood because O cells don't have any antigens and won't be automatically detected as "foreigners."

The second set of tests match tissue and serum. Human tissue may have up to twelve common antigens; the more the donor and recipient have in common, the better. Serum testing checks to ensure that the recipient's blood serum doesn't contain antibodies against the donor cells by mixing the two together and observing the outcome. The antibodies that attach to the cells are detected with fluorescence. If there are high quantities of antibodies, the donor cell gets destroyed, an indication that the donor and recipient do not match. The number of antibodies in serum fluctuates, so this test is run multiple times leading up to the donation, even if an earlier test has confirmed compatibility.

While waiting for a donor kidney, the potential recipient needs to stay healthy and to live as well as possible with a deteriorating kidney, in order to have the best chances in case a kidney becomes available.[49] The potential recipient needs to follow the nutritional plan, exercise regularly when possible,

---

48. Annette M. Jackson & Ed Kraus, "Blood Tests for Transplant," *National Kidney Foundation*, https://www.kidney.org/atoz/content/BloodTests-for-Transplant.

49. Danielle Peabody & Janelle Gonyea, "What you can do while waiting for the call," *National Kidney Foundation*, https://www.kidney.org/transplantation/transaction/TC/spring11/TCspring11_WaitingCall.

take all necessary medications, and attend doctors' visits, to keep the body functioning at its best.

There is no one standard path for families in need of a kidney for their loved one. They need, above all, open communication, patience, and an overabundance of love. Meanwhile, I hope the guidance given here can, in some small way, help family members figure out how to navigate this very difficult path. I strongly suggest getting advice from a sympathetic doctor and consulting with representatives of nonprofits dedicated to healing sufferers of kidney disease. Everyone wants to work in the best interest of the recipient. Kidney disease is an agonizing ordeal for all involved; the sooner a patient is healed, the closer that individual is to living fully again. Lean on family, lean on friends, and even lean on the kindness of strangers. The goal is always the same: to heal the suffering and bring this world closer to repair as well.[50]

A Vision for National Health Care in America

Concepts and values inherent in *halakhah* (Jewish law) have much to say about society's need to create a workable, sustainable health care financing system. One of the twentieth century's foremost rabbinic scholars in the area of medicine and *halakhah*, Rabbi Shlomo Zalman Auerbach, reminds us that everyone has the obligation to pay for the cure of a person who has a life-threatening illness: "From the straightforward reading of [BT] Sanhedrin 73a, we see that one is obligated to do everything to save him, and if not, one transgresses the negative commandment: 'Do not stand idly by the blood of your neighbor.'"[51]

---

50. Repairing the world itself is a most important Jewish value, known in Hebrew as *tikkun olam*.
51. Rabbi Shlomo Zalman Auerbach, *Minchat Shlomo*, V. 2, 86:4. The verse is Vayikra 19:16.

In a related ruling, classical Jewish law also states that physicians must not refrain from treating indigent patients: "[T]he Torah has given permission to doctors to heal. And it is a *mitzvah*. And it is included in 'saving a life.' And if a doctor refrains from healing it is as if he spilled blood."[52]

Centuries ago, Jewish communities in Europe embodied these values as they began to develop health care institutions. In the high Middle Ages, Jewish communities in Europe had begun creating a type of institution called a *hekdesh*,[53] that functioned both as an inn and as a place where sick travelers could receive rudimentary treatment.[54] With the beginning of the Jewish Enlightenment (in the eighteenth century) came the establishment of charitable organizations that ran hospitals for needy Jews throughout Europe. And in the United States, Jewish communities set up Jewish hospitals to serve a variety of needs that shifted with the times: to provide employment for Jewish doctors who faced discrimination elsewhere, to provide health care services to Jews who wished to be cared for in a Jewish environment, and to provide a mechanism for Jewish communities to help the general population.[55]

Outside of the Jewish world, governments across the globe have adopted a variety of health care funding mechanisms. In Europe, for example, countries have implemented different

---

52. *Shulchan Aruch Yoreh Deah* 336:1

53. The term *hekdesh* is the Hebrew for "holy purpose." This same term is used in the Talmud for donations to the Temple, indicating the esteem and value of these European institutions in the eyes of the creators.

54. The information about the *hekdesh* appears in the entry "Hospitals" of Encycopedia.com. https://www.encyclopedia.com/medicine/divisions -diagnostics-and-procedures/medicine/hospital.

55. See also Kottek, Samuel S., "The Hospital in Jewish History." Reviews of Infectious Diseases, vol. 3, no. 4, 1981, pp. 636–639. JSTOR, https:// www.jstor.org/stable/4452590.

health care financing programs in which the government mandates and pays for health care coverage.

Some use a single-payer approach in which the government acts as insurer – sometimes the only one – while private hospitals and doctors provide health care; some use universal coverage systems in which the government serves as both insurer and provider; and some require that individuals be covered by insurance but leave insurance options and health care details to the private sector.[56]

While European countries have implemented a variety of methods to achieve universal coverage, America struggles to find an approach. America searches for a means – and argues about the attempt – to cover every citizen. The first significant modern call for health insurance in the United States came in the early 1900s from the American Association of Labor Legislation (AALL).[57] In 1915, the AALL developed a bill that would have given health insurance to poor workers, supported by payments from the workers themselves, their employers, and the government. At the time, the American Medical Association (AMA) supported the bill, but organized labor did not, based on fears that the bill would, by protecting non-unionized workers, weaken unions; the effort faded by the beginning of World War I.

A political generation later, Franklin D. Roosevelt pushed New Deal initiatives that would spur the economy and protect the majority of those affected by the Great Depression. While the New Deal engendered significant progress for certain forms

---

56. David Rook, *How Does Healthcare in Europe Work?* JP Griffin Group (Jan. 11, 2018), https://www.griffinbenefits.com/employeebenefitsblog/how-does-healthcare-in-europe-work.

57. "A Brief History: Universal Health Care Efforts in the US," *Physicians for a National Health Program,* https://pnhp.org/a-brief-history-universal-health-care-efforts-in-the-us/.

of economic safety – Social Security, for example – it did not succeed with national health insurance. The Wagner-Murray-Dingell bill, which would have created a national health insurance plan financed by a payroll tax, did not gain traction in Congress when introduced in 1943, and the United States' involvement in World War II further stymied discussion of national coverage. The labor shortage during the war, however, spurred employers to attach health insurance options to employment packages.

The next major push for national health care came in 1945, shortly after the war ended. President Harry S. Truman proposed a tax on workers to pay for a national health insurance plan that would provide adequate medical care to all Americans.[58] President Truman understood that, without insurance, Americans "cannot afford[59] to pay...on an individual basis at the time they need it." Medical expenses could at any moment constitute a danger for the poor, but also "for a large proportion of normally self-supporting persons."

Though President Truman stressed that he was not proposing a government takeover of medical care, he faced an uphill battle. The AMA attacked the proposal, calling the Truman administration "followers of the Moscow party line" with "socialized medicine." Truman shot back to the AMA asking whether it was "un-American to visit the sick, aid the afflicted or comfort the dying?" President Truman could never overcome the strong opposition to the plan, however, and the effort to insure national health care stalled.

While Truman struggled to find a path forward toward na-

---

58. Howard Markel, "69 years ago, a president pitches his idea for national health care," *PBS*, https://www.pbs.org/newshour/health/november-19-1945-harry-truman-calls-national-health-insurance-program.
59. Emphasis mine.

tional health care, internationally other nations were strengthening their internal health care systems. In 1948, the Labour government in the United Kingdom established the National Health Service, which introduced universal health care. Every legal resident became eligible to register for the service, which made most medical care "free at point of use." The service also subsidizes prescriptions, optical and dental services, limiting the costs, and even making these services free for low-income residents. Nationwide taxes based on income cover the costs of the National Health Service.[60] Today, the National Health Service provides care for 65 million people. Similarly, in 1971, Canada established universal hospital and doctor care for all.[61]

It wasn't until 1965 that President Lyndon B. Johnson made the next serious attempt to establish universal health care coverage in the United States. As part of his Great Society initiative, Johnson got Medicare and Medicaid enacted, providing health care for the elderly and many poor Americans (with by-then-former President Harry Truman being issued the first Medicare card). But though Johnson achieved progress, national health insurance still proved elusive.

Decades passed with little movement for health care progress. When President Bill Clinton presented a comprehensive plan for health care financing in 1993, the plan got tepid support from key Democrats and hostile opposition from Republicans, who forcefully killed the prospects for national health care.[62] Between welfare reform by the Clinton Administration,

---

60. *England* NHS, https://www.england.nhs.uk/ourwork/.

61. Lorne Brown & Doug Taylor, "The Birth of Medicare," *Canadian Dimension,* https://canadiandimension.com/articles/view/the-birth -of-medicare.

62. Adam Clymer, Robert Pear & Robin Toner, "THE HEALTH CARE DEBATE: What Went Wrong? How the Health Care Campaign Collapsed – A special report.; For Health Care, Times Was A Killer," *The New York*

which did not try again to reform health care, and the second Bush Administration's focus on combatting terror, health care receded from the national agenda. Meanwhile, people continued to suffer from an endlessly complex, expensive, and often unfair web of ambiguous policies administered by the actuarial bureaucracy of health insurance companies. Charging extremely high rates, driving prices up, and refusing service to people with preexisting medical conditions, the companies provided little coverage for private individuals. Americans who had insurance for health care usually got it through their employers, or through government programs for the poor (Medicaid) or for the elderly (Medicare).[63] Many Americans remained without coverage, or without reliable coverage – a situation which could prove extremely costly or even deadly.

Finally, after years of stagnation, Congress passed President Barack Obama's imperfect, but workable, Patient Protection and Affordable Care Act (known as ACA or Obamacare) in 2010. The legislation sought to eliminate many significant health care exclusions, such as denying coverage to people with preexisting medical conditions (about half of Americans), setting annual or lifetime limits on coverage, not covering preventive care, and canceling policies when consumers became chronically ill. The underlying logic and premise of the ACA mandated that every person have insurance. The goal of including this mechanism was achieved in part by expanding Medicaid and creating exchanges where consumers could buy more

Times, https://www.nytimes.com/1994/08/29/us/health-care-debate-what-went-wrong-health-care-campaign-collapsed-special-report.html?pagewanted=all.

63. Louise Norris, "Are Health Insurance Companies Making Unreasonable Profits?" Verywellhealth.com, https://www.verywellhealth.com/health-insurance-companies-unreasonable-profits-1738941.

affordable insurance than before, since the ACA levied a tax on insurance companies, medical device companies, and individuals making more than $250,000 annually.[64] The designers hoped that this program would provide coverage to most of the Americans – nearly 50,000,000 – who lacked insurance.[65] The program succeeded in this partial goal. According to the United States Census Bureau, "In 2018, [only] 8.5 percent of people, or 27.5 million, did not have health insurance at any point during the year."[66]

The United States continues its decades-long raging debate about health care financing. American citizens, especially America's Jews and others who care about kidney health, need a speedy resolution to the problem of choosing a method for providing health care for all Americans.

National health care is vitally important for those with kidney disease. A life-and-death issue for those with kidney disease is coverage for people with preexisting conditions. Before Congress passed the ACA in 2014, insurance companies were allowed to deny coverage to people with preexisting conditions.[67] Since then, members of Congress have made frequent attempts to repeal this decision. A national health care system that covers everyone, regardless of their medical history, is crucial for

---

64. Noam N. Levey & Kyle Kim, "A side-by-side comparison of Obamacare and the GOP's replacement plans," *Los Angeles Times,* https://www.latimes.com/projects/la-na-pol-obamacare-repeal/.

65. https://www.healthreformvotes.org/congress/roll-call-votes/s396-111.2009.

66. Edward R. Berchick, Jessica C. Barnett, and Rachel D. Upton, "Health Insurance Coverage in the United States: 2018" NOVEMBER 08, 2019. Census Bureau REPORT NUMBER P60–267 (RV). Introduction.

67. "Pre-Existing Conditions," *U.S. Department of Health and Human Services,* https://www.hhs.gov/healthcare/about-the-aca/pre-existing-conditions/index.html.

the lives of people living with significant health conditions. For people with kidney disease, paying for dialysis three times a week – vital for their survival – would be disastrously costly, even for those who are financially well off. Without insurance, a dialysis patient would spend roughly $90,000 on hemodialysis, or about $50,000 on peritoneal dialysis, each year.

Kidney disease does not discriminate based on income. National health care could ensure that everyone receives their complete treatment, and that they can initiate treatment promptly. Without health insurance, patients might delay visiting a medical professional, thereby further delaying diagnosis and treatment – and putting their health at greater risk.

At the time of this writing, progress toward establishing national health care to cover all Americans is stymied by a rightward lurch in the highest levels of government. Powerful political leaders are totally hostile to any system providing the most fundamental health coverage. It feels endlessly frustrating for us to see elected officials – whose duties include promoting the general welfare of the nation – renege on their oath of office. Because of their hostility to health insurance, political leaders could at any moment sever the lifeline that sustains countless people. If our generation cannot achieve universal health insurance, then future generations of Americans will be left with the task.

Someday we will enact a grand vision of equal access to health care coverage. Ensuring that all people have the same access to health care is a moral objective that should not be limited by politics. Universal health care, though an enormous undertaking, is an imperative, for both the physical and spiritual health of our nation. May we only have the foresight and strength to see it made tangible for the countless people who struggle every day to fulfill their potential in this world.

This matters for Jews: the Jewish people are taught to have

compassion for those from all walks of life. When guests came to Abraham's tent, he didn't shun them even though they were strangers (Genesis 18:1). Caring for them might have seemed a burden to him. Instead, Abraham gave them utmost attention, preparing drinks and food for them and attending to their needs. These men, perhaps angels in the appearance of men, told him that his long-barren wife would have a child. Apparently, Abraham and Sarah were quick to care for strangers, and were therefore worthy of God's special attention due to this humanitarian concern.

We are to follow the path of the first chosen Jew by loving the stranger and ensuring that not only our family members but all people in society have access to basic health care protections. The ancient rabbis teach Jews the sanctity of human life in these words: " ...the first human being was created alone to teach that all who destroy a single life are as though they destroyed an entire universe, and those who save a single life are as if they had saved an entire universe."[68]

---

68. Jerusalem Talmud, Sanhedrin 4:22. Mishnah Sanhedrin 4:5; incidentally, the same sentence appears later in the Quran 5:32.

Chapter 6

Advocacy

Exploring Policy Issues

We badly need more donated kidneys. Should we start paying for them?

The need for living kidney donors is dire. Each year, thousands of Americans die while waiting for a kidney transplant.

I was privileged to be able to donate a kidney to a stranger who desperately needed one when I decided I could not morally justify living luxuriously with a backup kidney when someone else would die without my help. I felt compelled, both by my religion[1] and by my conscience, to sacrifice whatever I could to save another life. The procedure worked, and I am no worse for wear.

I was not financially compensated for my deed (nor would I want to be). But the truth is that a well-regulated market which offers financial incentives could save the lives of countless people. While kidney sales are illegal, they still occur; but they

---

1. The Jewish religion does not require one to specifically donate a kidney; however, saving life in general is, as we discussed earlier, a Jewish value and a biblical mandate.

occur underground,[2] which drives the price up substantially. The illegal market, inherently unregulated and unsupervised, rewards people who have connections or wealth, and causes terrible harm to the world's most vulnerable people. Bringing kidney sales out from the shadows could solve both of these problems, by increasing the supply of kidneys at a reasonable price and by safeguarding the easily exploitable poor.

Impoverished people sell their kidneys because they need the money, but the brokers who arrange the sale rarely inform the donors of the risks, and can get away with minimal compensation. Sometimes brokers lie, and promise that the kidney will grow back. Sometimes the brokers do not pay at all, as the donors have no way to enforce an illegal contract. The World Health Organization estimates that broker-purchased kidneys go for about $5,000, and are in turn sold to wealthy recipients for up to $200,000. The system exploits impoverished donors and rewards the brokers. The current unregulated and illegal network is abusive.

The Nepalese village of Hokse, near Kathmandu, is a heart-rending example.[3] It is known as "Kidney Village," since organ brokers have persuaded so many villagers to go to southern India, where they then sell a kidney to a foreigner to raise funds to pay debts or to support their families. Geeta, 37, mother of four, sold one of her kidneys for the measly sum of $2,000; she used the funds to buy a small house for her family. Her pain was for naught: In April 2015, the earthquake that struck Nepal levelled her modest home. Her family now lives in a structure made of corrugated iron and clear plastic wrap.

---

2. https://www.theguardian.com/world/2012/may/27/kidney-trade-illegal-operations-who.

3. http://www.dailymail.co.uk/news/article-3155817/Nepalese-village-sold-kidneys-organ-traffickers-buy-house-destroyed-devastating-earthquake.html.

In this worst of all possible worlds, kidney donors can gain only black-market incentives, and yet underground organ sales continue to happen en masse. We need a deep change. How can we transform this industry into one that ensures the health of the donor? What could protect potential donors from exploitive coercion? How can we eliminate exorbitant profit opportunities for organ brokers? Can we level the playing field to distribute the donated organs fairly?[4] Those who support the prohibition of incentives to donate assume that prohibition prevents abusive coercion to donate for profit. But like the prohibition of sex work, the prohibition of incentives to donate has failed. Miserably.

Banning organ sales may stop the exploiter if we enforce the ban vigorously enough, but it does nothing to help the exploited. We do not ban undignified work, perhaps, cynically, because we benefit from the people who do that work; or perhaps, idealistically, because we honor the agency of those who choose that work as their best option. If we succeed in banning undignified work, and organ sales, to protect the poor, we may also shut out the poor from their most realistic options. Rather than strive for moral purity for the most privileged, we should strive to save lives for, and the dignity of, the most underprivileged.

Though it would be nice if everyone would donate a kidney altruistically, we don't live in a utopia. And why should society require pure motives from one willing to take a health risk to save another's life? We don't expect pure altruism when paying firefighters and police officers. We pay soldiers to fight wars, doctors to treat ill patients, and researchers to work in labs handling the Ebola virus. So why should we be troubled by a penurious person getting paid for taking a small medical risk

---

4. https://www.theguardian.com/society/organ-donation.

that might save someone else's life? The mortality rate for kidney donation is less than that of non-essential plastic surgery.

As a rabbi – and as a human being who believes in the infinite dignity of the other – I believe saving human life is of utmost consequence. If most people will not donate altruistically, then we should embrace incentivizing people by offering them compensation and benefits. We must correct today's exploitative underground trafficking in vital organs. We must bring sanity to a system that lacks sanity. In doing so, we can save countless lives.

Incentivizing Organ Donation

When we pass from this world to the unknown realm of death and the afterlife, how do we wish to be remembered? Do we merely wish for our donations to earn recognition by having our names inscribed on physical monuments, perhaps on a bench in Central Park or on a concert hall, maybe even on a *beit midrash* (Jewish study hall)? Or, in that same spirit of postmortem generosity, do we wish to bequeath the gift of life to others? The challenges of kidney donation in particular form a subset of the broader question: How can we make organs available at rates both necessary and attainable?

The Imperative to Save a Life

How do we approach organ donation to be consistent with Jewish ideals? According to the Talmud, saving a life supersedes almost all other values, so organ donation should be recognized as one of the most noble religious acts according to Jewish law.

A source of the Jewish imperative to save the life of another[5]

---

5. But in the case of organ donation from a cadaver, whose mitzvah is it? Does the donor deserve the credit, or the bystanders? Rabbi Eliezer

appears in the Torah: "Do not stand idly by the blood of your fellow."[6]

The Talmudic rabbis taught that one is obligated to expend one's own resources to preserve the life of another.[7] Rabbi Yehezkel Landau of Prague (1713–93) taught that saving a life is such a righteous priority that it overrides the prohibitions against cutting into or desecrating a cadaver:

> But I question: If this case were to be labeled even possible lifesaving, then why do you need all the arguments back and forth? After all, it is clearly laid out and specifically stated that even possible lifesaving pushes aside Shabbat observance, which is a weighty matter [and therefore unquestionably "degrading" the dead would be permitted].[8]

Two Primary Objections to Organ Donation

Opponents of organ donation among religious Jews commonly

Waldenberg and Rabbi Yitzchak Yaakov Weiss, twentieth century halachic authorities, argue that it cannot be the mitzvah of the deceased, since a dead individual is not obligated to save a life (or perform do any other mitzvot). Though one has no obligations after death, we may all have the obligation to put the right orders in place while we are alive, and the bystanders may have the obligation to intervene to carry out the orders of the deceased (Tzitz Eliezer 13:91; Minhat Yitzhak 5:8). However, an individual has no legal authority after he or she dies, and the survivors do not necessarily have to follow the will. Even so, we do generally follow the principle that it is a mitzvah *lekayeim divrei hameit* (we are to honor the words of the deceased) unless the requests are immoral.

6. Leviticus 19:16
7. Babylonian Talmud Sanhedrin 73a
8. Noda bi'Yehuda (vol. 2, Yoreh Deah 210). To be fair, Rabbi Landau was speaking in theory. In practice, he did not think what the medical school in London was doing should be considered lifesaving. For more on this, see the first essay in Zev Farber and Irving (Yitz) Greenberg, "Extending the Definition of Lifesaving."

put forward two main objections to the practice. First, they say that a person buried without a certain organ will be resurrected in the World to Come without that organ.[9] Second, removing an organ for donation is a violation of the dignity or sanctity of the human corpse.[10]

Regarding the first point, admittedly a handful of authorities make such a claim, such as Rabbi Yeshua Shimon Haim Ovadia[11] and Rabbi Ovadia Hedaya. Nevertheless, no less an authority than former Chief Sephardic Rabbi of Israel Ovadia Yosef wrote that such a claim has little if any basis in traditional sources and makes little sense.[12] Classical legal texts such as Maimonides' *Mishneh Torah* and the *Shulchan Aruch* do not claim that one must be buried with all of one's organs to be resurrected whole. Therefore, performing this mitzvah yields only spiritual gain, not loss.

As for the second point, that removing the organs from a corpse violates the body, to my mind nothing can be further from the truth.[13] If anything, by taking the deceased person's organs and using them to save another's life, we involve the donor in one last mitzvah, *piku'ah nefesh* (saving a life), and quite an important one at that.

---

9. And, specifically in regard to kidneys, if only one kidney is necessary, it shouldn't make a whole lot of difference if one is missing in the World to Come.

10. Violating the sanctity of the human corpse is referred to in Hebrew as *bizui hameit* (disgracing the deceased).

11. Yismach Levav, Yoreh Deah 45. Rabbi Ovadia (20th century, Morocco) served as the rabbi of Sefrou, Morocco.

12. Yabi'a Omer, vol. 8 Hoshen Mishpat 11. For more on this, see the third essay in Zev Farber and Irving (Yitz) Greenberg, "Extending the Definition of Lifesaving," in *Halakhic Realities: Collected Essays on Organ Donation.*

13. This is my view, but for an alternative one, see Nehemia Polen's essay "Personal Identity in Death: An Aggado-Halakhic Critique."

Piku'ah Nefesh: *A Central Commandment*

In the past, failure of the heart, liver, kidneys, or any other vital organ, meant death; but that is no longer true. The medical miracle of organ donation has changed all that. Most organ recipients live many years after transplant.[14] To state the obvious, however, for organ donation to be effective, organs need to be available to give to patients in need.

The situation is quite dire:

In the United States, the number of kidney transplants, which represent about five-sixths of all organ transplants, remained static for a decade at 16,000 to 17,000 a year, but has steadily climbed in the last several years to around 21,000 a year. Meanwhile, the waiting list for kidneys from deceased donors has nearly doubled, passing 120,000 in in recent years. The median wait time for an adult is more than four years, and more than 4,000 die waiting each year.[15]

Consider the utter desperation experienced by thousands of Americans currently on a waiting list for organs, a waiting list that leads to success slowly or not at all. The waiting list grows by four thousand every day, as the population ages and as more people suffer from hypertension, type 2 diabetes, and other diseases.[16] In 2020 in the United States, 91,099 kidney transplants were needed; only 22,817 were available. Tens of thousands of others wait for bone, cartilage, skin, and heart valve transplants. Each organ donor has the capacity, after death,

---

14. See the U.S. Department of Health and Human Services' organ donor "about" page, https://www.organdonor.gov/learn/organ-donation-statistics and https://data.hrsa.gov/topics/health-systems/organ-donation.

15. https://www.iowadonornetwork.org/understanding-donation/current-statistics

16. See the WebMD entry on Organ Donation and Transplant. http://www.webmd.com/a-to-z-guides/organ-donation-facts.

to clear eight people off of the organ transplant waiting list and to help as many as fifty people through donation of corneas, bone, tendons, cartilage, heart valves, skin and more.

Here are some sobering statistics:[17]

- There are currently well over 100,000 people awaiting life-saving organ transplants in the U.S. Of these, 85% are waiting for kidney transplants.
- In 2020, 21,656 kidney transplants took place in the U.S. Deceased donors accounted for over 11,000 transplants; fewer than 5,000 transplants came from living donors.
- Someone is added to the organ-transplant waiting list every nine minutes.
- Every day, 17 people die while waiting for a lifesaving organ transplant.

Incentives for Organs

For the medical, economic, and moral well-being of our society, I believe that countries should adjust their organ donation requirements to incentivize organ donations; this, too, is a mandate of the highest order and falls under the rubric of *piku'ah nefesh*.

To draw in the more than 140 million other citizens who have refused or just neglected to state their preference to donate, we may need to creatively provide reasons for people to choose to become organ donors. Furthermore, it is important to make sure that people who wish to donate make their intentions known to family members (or another guardian) well in advance. Too often, families fail to have these crucial conversations and there is ambiguity, even conflict, as to whether

---

17. See https://optn.transplant.hrsa.gov/data/; https://data.hrsa.gov/topics/health-systems/organ-donation; https://www.organdonor.gov/learn/organ-donation-statistics.

an individual's organs should be donated. Leaving instructions in a will is often insufficient, as the decision to retrieve organs usually must be made before any will is found or read after death.[18]

Ways of Incentivizing Organ Donation

A number of methods have been proposed to maximize and encourage organ donation. Some programs currently are in use; others are merely proposals that have been discussed:

Opt-out. Most of the United States has an opt-in system, where people are not donors unless they specifically request to be organ donors, through organ donor cards or through filling out a form when renewing a driver's license.[19] Several European countries and Singapore have an opt-out system, in which everyone is an organ donor unless he or she has specifically requested not to be a donor.[20]

Belgium and Austria, for example, use an opt-out system and have experienced tremendous success. More than 95% of those countries' citizens are donors, meaning that fewer than 5 percent have used the opt-out system to state their unwillingness to donate, allowing for many more donations.

Nevertheless, in my view, outside authorities (government, medical management, etc.) cannot and should not override the will of the deceased's family. If the deceased has not made a formal legal commitment to donate, then the choice should rest

---

18. See the discussion on the U.S. Legal Wills question and answer page on organ donation. http://www.uslegalwills.com/organ_donation.

19. See Jahel Queralt Lange, "Hypothetically Donated Organs," Practical Ethics: Ethics in the News (2010), http://blog.practicalethics.ox.ac.uk/2011/01/hypothetically-donated-organs/.

20. These issues also are discussed in Noam Zohar, "Is Our Public Policy on Brain Death Ethical?" *Halakhic Realities: Collected Essays on Brain Death,* 393–98.

with the family. There always is and always should be a balance between individual autonomy and the public interest.[21]

Mandated choice. A similar system, a version of which has been tried in Illinois, is mandated choice, in which adults must choose whether they will be organ donors.[22] The choice takes place at certain official points, such as when people renew drivers' licenses, and is legally binding. Illinois' method has had great success, and the state boasts a 60% donor rate, nearly double the average American rate.

Financial incentives. Other proposals grant incentives to those who agree to become organ donors; for example, creating a market system that pays donors for non-essential organs (e.g., for kidneys).[23] This need not be only a cash payment: We might consider a tax credit, a retirement contribution, earlier access to Medicare, and similar benefits.

Priority to donors and their families. Another approach prioritizes those who have agreed to be organ donors to receive organs if and when they should develop the need. Israel uses such a plan.[24]

---

21. In the United States, one has the right to offer a body for organ donation, but one cannot be forced – by a hospital, let's say – to allow organs to be removed. Imagine if the government were to require all corpses to undergo autopsies or pass legislation requiring that all bodies be cremated. Such exercise of power would be catastrophic; we must always remain diligent in preserving the familial intimacy and religious practices of such important and emotional decisions.

22. See Richard H. Thaler, "Opting In vs. Opting Out?" *New York Times* (September 26, 2009), http://www.nytimes.com/2009/09/27/business/economy/27view.html?_r=0.

23. See Thaler, "Opting In."

24. See Danielle Ofri, "In Israel, a New Approach to Organ Donation," *New York Times* Blogs (February 16, 2012), http://well.blogs.nytimes.com/2012/02/16/ in-israel-a-new-approach-to-organ-donation/.

Procurement agencies. The United States has made positive strides in increasing organ donation by setting up organ procurement agencies and bone marrow registries, and through these efforts has registered 145 million Americans to donate their organs.[25] While that statistic seems impressive, it also reveals that this opt-in system has resulted in only a little over half of Americans offering to serve as organ donors.

Ease of registration. Easier methods could enable potential donors to register their wishes clearly, possibly through social media or a special website or iPhone and Android applications.

Government-controlled buying. Iran, certainly no role-model nation, is the only country to pay residents for their organs and also the only country to have virtually no waiting list.[26] Although it is less than ideal, compensation – in a controlled and regulated market – may be a path to consider going forward to ensure that we can save lives.

Problems with Incentives

The idea of a market system for paying donors has been met with resistance due to the belief that it would primarily benefit the wealthy, who could offer the highest bids for organs.[27]

Worldwide, about 200,000 people are on waiting lists for kidneys, and ominously, about 10% of kidney transplants involve

---

25. See the U.S. Department of Health and Human Services' organ donor legislation history page. https://www.organdonor.gov/about-us/legislation-policy/history and "Organ Donation Statistics," U.S. Department of Health and Human Services. https://www.organdonor.gov/learn/organ-donation-statistics.gov/statistics-stories/statistics.htm.
26. See Ahad J. Ghods and Shekoufeh Savaj, "Iranian Model of Paid and Regulated Living – Unrelated Kidney Donation," *Clinical Journal of the American Society of Nephrology* (2006). http://cjasn.asnjournals.org/content/1/6/1136.full.
27. See Thaler, "Opting In," note 22.

payment to a non-relative of another nationality, which suggests that many poor people are selling their organs for money.[28] According to the World Health Organization, thousands of people a year in India, Pakistan, the Philippines, China, and other countries sell their organs to mostly wealthy recipients, in spite of international efforts to prohibit these activities.[29]

Transplants brokered on underground, illegal markets are often accessible only to the wealthiest individuals: *The New York Times* found that in recent years brokers typically have charged clients $100,000 to $200,000 to cover expenses associated with a transplant.[30]

Such outlandish prices for organs are directly related to the rampant problem of organ trafficking. As the legal market continues to struggle to obtain a supply of healthy organs from willing donors, organ cartels ruthlessly bully vulnerable people to part with their organs for little recompense. Though they are criminalized across the globe, organ cartels exert an increasingly influential force in developing countries. In 2008, a worldwide conference of transplant practitioners handed the organ trade an unequivocal rebuke. The group's manifesto, called the Declaration of Istanbul, asserted that trafficking

---

28. About seventy-five nations have programs for the deceased to donate their organs. Oddly, neither Canada nor Russia has a national organization that coordinates transplants, while in South America and most of North Africa and Asia, national governmental or non-governmental organizations are responsible for organ transplants.

29. See Yosuke Shimazono, "The State of the International Organ Trade: A Provisional Picture Based on Integration of Available Information," *Bulletin of the World Health Organization*. https://apps.who.int/iris/bitstream /handle/10665/269908/PMC2636295.pdf?sequence=1&isAllowed=y.

30. See Kevin Sack, "Transplant Brokers in Israel Lure Desperate Kidney Patients to Costa Rica," *New York Times* (August 17, 2014), http://www .nytimes.com/2014/08/17/world/middleeast/transplant-brokers-in-israel -lure-desperate-kidney-patients-to-costa-rica.html.

violated "the principles of equity, justice, and respect for human dignity, and should be prohibited."[31] The declaration did not succeed. The market for trafficked kidneys grows unabated, as the gap between supply and demand widens each year. If more organs were available, the demand to buy organs from poor people would be substantially alleviated. We now need to reconsider our idealistic plan of relying exclusively on altruistic donations.

We need to convince more people to sign up as organ donors, even if it means paying them. Legal kidney donations meet only 10% of the demand.[32] We dare not be so concerned with the purity of our motives that we condemn humans to needless premature death. In a legal market, we could try to limit exploitation of the poor. We do not have to solve all the problems of organ donation by designing a perfect system all at once. We can experiment with new programs, carefully monitor their effectiveness, and modify them as needed, to produce a better result than is our current practice.

Why People Object to Donating: The Need for Better Education

One British study indicated that about 30% of relatives refused to allow organs from their brain-dead family members to be retrieved, even to save the lives of others.[33] The families raised two objections: their fear that the organ will be removed before death (i.e., that brain death is a part of the process of dying

---

31. For details, see "The Declaration of Istanbul on Organ Trafficking and Transplant Tourism," http://www.declarationofistanbul.org/.
32. See Shimazono, "The state of the international organ trade . . ." note 29.
33. See Paul Gill and Ian Hulatt, "Relatives' Refusal in Organ Donation: 'It's Mostly a Matter of Respect,'" *Nursing in Critical Care* 5.5 (2000): 236–239, http://www.academia.edu/817382/Relatives_refusal_in_organ_donation_its_mostly_a_matter_of_respect.

but is not yet the finality of death), and that the body will be mutilated during the process. Some also voiced that the person "has been through enough." A Gallup poll taken thirty years ago found that 20% of people objected to the idea that they would be "cut up after they died."[34]

To assuage the fears of patients and their families, a team including nurses, physicians, other hospital staff, and clergy, could provide reassuring emotional support and factual instruction, showing that the organ will be removed only after death, and that the body will be treated with the utmost respect. Even with the best instructional efforts, we can anticipate that some families will still remain unalterably opposed to donation. While there tends to be consensus regarding organ donation among the major religions, there are some groups and religions (e.g., Roma and Shinto) whose beliefs are incompatible with organ donation.

Taking but Not Giving: The Israeli Policy and the Unfortunate Circumstances that Brought it About

Certain groups of Jews have argued for allowing Jews to *receive* organs removed from people who donated after brainstem death, but still forbidding Jews to *willingly donate* in the same circumstance.[35] This policy of taking but not giving is morally problematic, and it endangers Jews by further equipping people of hate. We cannot ignore the concern of *mishum eivah*, the halachic warning against acting in such a way as to cause gentiles to hate Jews. It would be understandable for the entire medical

---

34. See Gill and Hulatt, "Relatives' Refusal."

35. For a detailed discussion and critique of this stance, see Rabbi Eugene Korn's essay and Rabbi Joseph Telushkin's brief statement critiquing this practice, in *Halakhic Realities: Collected Essays on Organ Donation*, Koren: Jerusalem. 2017.

community to reject the "taking but not giving" approach, and to look askance at Jews who advocate for it.

Though a small segment of the Israeli population understood "taking but not giving" as a correct policy, other segments simply did not react at all to the option of donating organs. People generally followed the tradition of prompt intact burial, and did not consider donation. The organ donation rate in Israel remained unusually low. The situation had gotten so bad that Eurotransplant, the organization responsible for the allocation of donor organs to European countries, would no longer provide vital organs to Israel.

Lavee's Initiative: Getting Israel to Act against "Taking but not Giving"

In 2005, Dr. Jacob Lavee, director of the Heart Transplantation Unit at the Sheba Medical Center, Israel, operated to give heart transplants to two ultra-Orthodox patients, both of whom had informed him that they personally would not donate their organs but would accept organs from others. Dr. Lavee regarded this position as unfair and inconsistent, so over the next several years he worked with medical, legal, academic, and religious authorities to change Israeli law.

Dr. Lavee's efforts achieved results: "In 2008, responding to a widening gap between need and availability of transplant organs, Israel's Ministry of Health adopted a program of incentivized cadaveric organ donation."[36] Israel organ transplants are given first to those who themselves have signed donor cards or who have relatives who have been donors. The government

---

36. Corinne Berzon, "Israel's 2008 Organ Transplant Law: continued ethical challenges to the priority points model" *Israel Journal of Health Policy Research* 2018, 7:11. https://www.ncbi.nlm.nih.gov/pmc/articles /PMC5855996/.

covers donors' expenses related to organ donation, and mandates the equivalent of forty days' pay to donors. Furthermore, Dr. Lavee achieved a consensus among all but the ultra-Orthodox community on a definition of brain death that makes organ donation possible, and an endorsement of organ donation as a reflection of the Talmudic principle that saving a life is more important than virtually any other consideration.

In response, the Israeli media began an education campaign to convey the message that Judaism does not ban – and even encourages – organ donation. Soon organ donor cards were issued at a rate about ten times higher than before the education campaign, and transplants rose by 60%.

In granting priority to people who have donated organs or even signed donor cards, Israel has become one of the first countries in the world to incorporate non-medical criteria in the organ donation system. Israel has implemented this law over the objections of some ethicists. Medical necessity remains, of course, the first priority in choosing recipients. So, regardless of their stance on organ donation, the ultra-Orthodox will continue to benefit while refusing to make donations themselves. Nevertheless, prioritizing potential donors is a step in the right direction: We must be a nation of givers, for this is the purpose of our people.

The Israeli government should continue to lead the way toward incentivizing organ donation. Israel is in desperate need of intervention, given its unfortunately low rate of organ donation from the deceased: "About 15% of Israeli adults are registered as donors, according to the Health Ministry's National Transplant Center, compared with nearly half in the United States."[37] However, the number of transplants performed in

---

37. See Kevin Sack, "A Clash of Religion and Bioethics Complicates Organ Donation in Israel," New York Times (August 17, 2014), http://

Israel continues to increase each year, with more families giving consent for their relatives' organs to be donated.[38] We hope that this trend will continue and that more people will register as organ donors in the future. In Israel as elsewhere, we need to teach people to donate, to do our part, and not just buy organs from impoverished donors in developing countries. Communities must step up for community members.

Concluding Imperative

Mature religious thinking requires that we consider the big picture, namely, our spiritual existence after our physical existence expires. This mature consideration requires that we have open and honest conversations with our loved ones about what we want to happen with our organs after we leave this world, even though these discussions may be emotionally charged and difficult.

www.nytimes.com/2014/08/17/world/middleeast/a-clash-of-religion
-and-bioethics-complicates-organ-donation-in-israel.html.

38. Ido Efrati, "Record High Number of Organ Transplants Made in Israel in 2018, Report Shows," *Haaretz* (January 16, 2019), https://www.haaretz.com/israel-news/.premium-record-high-number-of-organ-transplants-made-in-israel-in-2018-report-shows-1.6846700.

Chapter 7
Stories from other Rabbis and Jewish Educators (written in their own voice)

Dr. Erica Brown
Search My Heart (and My Kidneys)

We say repeatedly in our prayers on the Days of Awe that God is inspecting our hearts and our kidneys for wrongdoing. As a kidney donor, I prayed on those days that with only one kidney there was less to inspect! This strange notion finds confirmation in a Talmudic statement about King David, who cried out to God, "Examine me and subject me to an ordeal, as it says: 'Examine me, Lord, and subject me to an ordeal; try my kidneys and my heart.'"[1] Our Sages teach that a person has two kidneys for a reason: "One advises him to do good and one advises him to do evil."[2] I hoped that when my left kidney was removed, it would remove with it any desire to eat chocolate

---

1. Babylonian Talmud, Sanhedrin 107a
2. Babylonian Talmud, Berachot 61a

in the middle of the night and leave only wisdom in its place. No such luck!

In the ancient world, when anatomical knowledge was evolving, the kidneys were actually regarded as the brain is today. The kidneys were understood to be the seat of the emotions, one's energy and one's intelligence. This is reflected in a verse from one of the most philosophical of all biblical books: Job. "Who places wisdom in the kidneys, or who deposits understanding in the heart?"[3] In fact, kidneys are mentioned over thirty times in the Hebrew Bible, mostly in reference to sacrifices but also with regard to a body part that both preserves and exudes a special kind of knowledge. Rabbi Judah, one of the most famous Talmudic sages, said, "The kidneys advise, the heart understands, and the tongue shapes the voice that emerges."[4]

As a kidney donor, I've reflected on why the kidneys were associated with all of this goodness. I believe the reason is that the kidneys function as efficient filters for getting rid of waste and toxins, while returning vital substances into the bloodstream. It's a perfect spiritual metaphor for repentance. When it comes to transformational change, we need to minimize wrongdoing, strengthen what is currently working, and create good filters when we make daily decisions. That's a good reason to keep both kidneys.

But I was prepared to forego one. I thought about a kidney donation for many years and tried to donate one about five years before my actual operation. Generally, a number of people are tested at one time since it's not easy to find a perfect match. In that first instance, despite a few days of testing, the person in need received a kidney from someone further along in the

---

3. Job 38:36
4. Babylonian Talmud, Shabbat 33b

testing process. Years later, I learned that a friend with a young family needed a new kidney before renal failure. I remember the exact moment when the nurse called to tell me that I did not match his blood type. I was crushed. But then she suggested a match. If I give my kidney to someone else with an A plus blood type, my friend who was an O blood type would receive a kidney within 14 days of needing one. My disappointment quickly turned into relief. If I couldn't give him my own kidney, I could at least expedite the long wait for him. In the state of Maryland, the average wait time is 3 to 5 years. In New York, it's longer. That's too long to wait for anyone with a serious health condition.

When I did the spiritual calculus as to whether or not to donate a kidney, the answer was obvious, at least for me. I went into education because I wanted to make a difference in people's actual lives. Sometimes that happens, but it's rare. Being a kidney donor was one way to very literally change the trajectory of someone's life. And despite a rather long process of recovery – I was out-and-about at 6 weeks but did not really feel myself until after 3–6 months – I still believe it was one of the best decisions I've ever made and would gladly do it again if I could.

As of this writing, it has been a year-and-a-half since my kidney donation. I have observed two Yom Kippur days of fasting where God introspected the one kidney I have left. And while I continue to make constant mistakes, inadvertently hurt people I love and ignore calls for justice, I joke that when carefully assessing my remaining kidney, God might excuse a lapse of judgment because I gave one kidney away. Rather than diminish wisdom, I think donating a kidney is a smart thing to do for a healthy person. I can function without one kidney while someone in the world cannot live without [even] one. It doesn't get more basic than that.

I don't know much about my recipient nor will I likely ever know. In order for us to make contact, a year must pass; both of us have to sign a document that we'd like to know the identity of the other. I signed. Perhaps he did not. Maybe he will feel better or less guilty about the surgery if he doesn't know who I am. That is his right, and I respect it. Although he is a stranger, we are all one existential family. And while people thought it odd to undergo such a difficult procedure for someone whose name I do not know, I found it to be the ultimate expression of my humanity.

A few days after the surgery, the transplant coordinator gave me a manila envelope that contained a simple note of a few sentences. It began with "Hello" on the top line. It continued in a very simple fashion: "I don't really know what to say except thank you. I wanted to let you know what a difference your kindness has made in my life." My recipient shared how much he has grown to appreciate life and not take it for granted, and then offered this prayer: "May God continue to bless you and your family." He told me that he would keep me in his "thoughts and prayers always." I wept when I read it. I have always believed in the kindness of strangers as an affirmation of hope. I am so grateful that on that day I could be that stranger for him. I still do not know his name.

At the time, my recipient was a 67-year-old resident of Wisconsin who received my left kidney as it was transported from Johns Hopkins on a summer day in mid-July. In a breathtaking miracle, my kidney left my body after a 3–4-hour surgery at about ten in the morning; it was packaged in ice and was flown commercially from Baltimore to Wisconsin (I hope it didn't get stuck in a middle seat!). Before that day was over, it gave someone else a new lease on life.

Like me, my recipient is the parent of four, as he shared with me in his anonymous post-op letter. Like me, he has two grandchildren. I am told that the kidney transplant was a success. I hope it enables him to spend quality time with his family without the dark cloud of kidney failure looming over him. While we do not know each other, we are linked forever through the surgeries that took place that day. When I was in recovery, a Hopkins' employee handed me a fleece blanket to use and take home that said, "Whoever saves one life, it is as if he has saved the world." It did not attribute the saying to the Talmud where it originated. But I smiled wide when I read it. Our Jewish wisdom had me quite literally covered, and for the first time in my life, I could truly and humbly say that I understood what that statement means.

Rabbi Aryeh Bernstein

On June 1, 2017, the 2nd day of Shavuot, I donated a kidney to a stranger. This enabled a friend-of-a-friend to receive a kidney at the same time, in the same operating room, from a different stranger, saving her life. Many people have asked me why I volunteered to do this. The simple answer is that this precious organ was the difference between life and death for someone else and was a spare part for me that cost me, in my particular situation, relatively little to rehouse. What follows is a more detailed and verbose version of that simple answer.

The Trivial, Personal Factors Keeping Us from Doing the Meaningful Things We Want to Do

Years ago, I first read about the advances in kidney transplant surgery and how remarkably low risk and high success a procedure it has become for donors. I do not remember when and where I learned about these advances nor about how demand for kidneys so grossly overwhelms the small number available, but for years, these basic facts have shaped my understanding of the necessity for many more people to donate kidneys. I have known people suffering kidney failure, including my grandmother of blessed memory, Esther Malkin Lesner, so, from a young age I have understood the severity of kidney failure, despite the wondrous technological advance of dialysis. Knowing that there are people at risk of dying and that I can help them seriously raise their chances of living at low risk to myself gnawed at me for years. I happen to be a person who is blessed not to be particularly afraid of hospitals, surgery, or general anesthesia. However, I am terrified of logistics, and for years, I put off looking into the practicalities of how to become a living donor and what's involved simply because, irrationally, I felt frozen before the prospect of a simple internet search, not knowing how procedurally complicated it might become.

The Teachers and Friends Guiding Us Across the Line

In 2012, my teacher, Dr. Devora Steinmetz, donated a kidney, and her article about it was very moving to me. A few years later, my friend, Rabbi Dr. Shmuly Yanklowitz, donated a kidney, and I had the privilege to be present at his provocative and inspiring ELI talk about that decision. Devora, Shmuly, and I are all different people. Our stories are different, our strengths, weaknesses, and vulnerabilities are different. But their words left deep impressions on me, arousing and animating with new urgency the general prospect of kidney donation, which had been whispering in my ear for years. Especially resonant for me was Devora's discussion of how different acts of *chesed* (kindness) can be easier or harder for different people, and her vigorous resistance to the notion that donating a kidney to a stranger is irrational or insufferably righteous. Her words helped me recognize my reactions to hearing about other people donating kidneys – *"I should really look into that"* – versus my reaction to hearing about friends rescuing animals from slaughter to raise and nurture in their homes – *"Wow, I'm so glad you're doing that; I could never do that."* Devora's words helped clarify for me that kidney donation is a significant thing to do, but it is also *normal*. Different people have different fears, resources, life circumstances, and abilities, according to which different potential deeds of kindness and life-giving can be, for one person, an extreme measure of piety and sacrifice; while for another it is in the realm of *mitzvah* – fulfilling the commandment to choose life. Kidney donation is not *objectively* extreme. It is *subjectively* so for some people, and I may not be one of those people.

Similarly, resonant to me was the core question Shmuly raised: In my life, have I given more or taken more? Like Shmuly, I found it completely and obviously clear to me in my own life that I have taken far, far more than I have given. I was moved to tears by the clip of him reflecting just before his surgery, "I can't imagine being on the other end and feeling like I was sick or dying and nobody cared." For my whole adult life I've been a Deadhead, a devoted fan of the band the Grateful Dead, and Shmuly's statement reminded me of a teaching of Grateful Dead bassist Phil Lesh. Lesh received a life-saving liver donation in 1998 from a young man named Cody, who was killed in a motor vehicle accident. Four months later, Lesh was back on stage and in every subsequent concert since, before the finale, Lesh speaks to his audience about the urgency of signing up to be an organ donor. In this teaching, known in Deadhead circles simply as the "Donor Rap," Lesh urges the audience members to commit to signing up for the donor registry and to tell their families and friends that they've done so. On some concert recordings, I have heard him add words that lodged a permanent home between my ears: "If you or someone you loved needed an organ, would you accept it? If so, it's only fair to be willing to donate." Just a few months before Shmuly's talk, I was fortunate enough to attend the Grateful Dead's 50-year anniversary concert at Soldier Field in Chicago. Lesh's Donor Rap reverberated in my head for months after that show. I began to see kidney donation as the realest translation of Deadhead culture and ethos: "Strangers stopping strangers just to shake their hand/Everybody is playing in a heart of gold band" (my favorite Dead song, "Scarlet Begonias"). Somebody needs a miracle, I have an extra, and I'm not using it. It should be theirs.

As Shmuly's talk was fresh in my mind, my dear friend and sister-in-law, Rabbi Lizzi Heydemann, posted on Facebook that a family friend and member of her remarkable spiritual community, Mishkan Chicago, was in need of a kidney donor. Here was an outstretched hand and a ramp for what felt like the hardest part for me. I told her to put us in touch. We met over lunch and she answered my most basic questions, including assuring me, since we're captive to the dystopic and cruel economy of the plutocracy that is the United States, that my mediocre insurance would not have to pay for anything. All I had to do to get the ball rolling was make one phone call to the transplant center number she gave me. After that, they reached out to me. I spent a good chunk of 2016 undergoing many rigorous screening tests at the University of Illinois at Chicago Medical Center, including consultations with the nephrologist, the surgeons, and social workers. While I was not a match for this new friend, UIC was able to arrange a double-match, so that simultaneously, the kidney in my body was transplanted to one person (who chose to remain anonymous), while a kidney from another donor (also unknown to me) was transplanted to Lizzi's friend, who, along with her mother, became my friend as well by the time of the surgery.

What Were the Factors that Made Kidney Donation Not Prohibitive for Me?

Physical Health

In my experience, prospective donors are not cleared if there are significant risks. The doctors, nurses, and social worker discussed various barriers to being a donor. Some of these had to do with physical health. I don't smoke, I drink only casually, I don't use drugs. I haven't had an STI, obesity has not been a factor in my life, and I don't have other physical health challenges which would sap my body of the resources it would need for a speedy and smooth recovery.

Emotional Experience Around Hospitals and Surgery

Another factor is one's emotional state. Some people may have great physical health but be terrified of hospitals, blood, or surgery. I'm not. Why? I don't know, but since I'm not, I felt a heightened sense of obligation to agree to this surgery, since other potential donors would face much more prohibitive fears and anxiety.

Support System I: Employment Structure

Other factors include one's support system. I was told that I would need a lot of support for the first two weeks after surgery and that I shouldn't expect to do much of any work during that period. After two weeks, I was told to expect to be able to work full time and resume life activities, but that I would still need community support, because I would be restricted from lifting more than ten pounds or engaging in other physical exertion until six weeks post-surgery. I understood that all sorts of other potential donors would fall out of the pool for these reasons. Perhaps they're perfectly healthy and comfortable with surgery, but their place of work would not accommodate them. My employers and colleagues at Avodah, the Jewish Council on Urban Affairs, and my co-teacher in the Hyde Park Teen Beit Midrash were fully encouraging and happy to cover me in work during the recuperation period. Perhaps someone has two weeks' vacation time, but their work involves athletics or physical labor, meaning that they would have to miss work for six weeks. I sit at a computer and teach classes. If all went well, I knew that I could expect to be [fully] back at work in two weeks. Perhaps a potential donor has young children who need to be carried and it's an undue burden on other childcare providers for a parent not to be able to lift their child for six weeks. I don't have children. Recognizing that none of the many factors which make kidney surgery an unreasonable sacrifice or impossibility applied to me amplified the sense of responsibility I had to make available the spare kidney housed in my body.

Support System 11: Who Are My Angels?

The transplant coordinators emphasized the importance of having a strong support system. I'm blessed to play in a huge, raucous, banging, heart of gold band in my life and knew that I would have abundant help healing. My retired mother, who lives just a couple of blocks away from me, was emphatic in her total support, adding that she had even considered kidney donation herself in the past, but had some technical obstacles. She encouraged me to recuperate in their home, where I would be cared for, fed, and provided with amenities. As an added bonus, she worked at the UIC Medical School for over a decade and was herself personally comfortable with that hospital and with hospitals in general. The last thing I would need on operation day would be to have to calm down a relative who accompanied me. My mother was calm, rational, and support-ive. I am also blessed to live in a real community, with webs of relationships, through synagogue and other affiliations. Friends, my partner, and relatives in and outside my neighborhood stepped up in support: bringing me food, carrying groceries, accompanying me on walks, and more. I knew I would not be alone and I turned out to be surrounded by all the practical and emotional support I could have hoped for and then some.

The Flowing Cycle of Teaching Torah

I was also buoyed by the wonderful students of the Hyde Park Teen Beit Midrash, with whom I had spent the year learning Talmudic wisdom about how the value of saving a life is fundamental to Jewish law, overriding even capital prohibitions (the 8th chapter of Tractate Yoma). My co-teacher, the brilliant young scholar-teacher Avital Morris, happily volunteered to teach solo for our final session of the year, as I recuperated and prepared to come home from the hospital. That night, one of the high school students and her mother came to fulfill the mitzvah of *bikkur cholim*/visiting the sick. Thalia taught me what they had learned in the Beit Midrash that morning – a halakhic responsum of the late Rav Ovadia Yosef on the propriety of organ donation, translating the same early texts we had studied all year into this immediately relevant scenario. I had thought a lot about how my donation of a kidney would, with the help of God, save a life; and, in this case, participate in saving two lives, because of the double-transplant. I had not thought about how the experience would deepen or proliferate Torah learning, leading to the most precious experience a teacher can have: being taught Torah by my student. *Mitzvah goreret mitzvah!* Fulfillment of one sacred commandment leads to another![5] The poetry of participating in this transplant on Shavuot, the holiday of the reception of Torah, and such experiences of amplified generosity and interconnectedness,

---

5. Mishnah Pirkei Avot 4:2

brought to life a *midrash*[6] shared with me by my friend Shira
Ben-Sasson days before the transplant:

"…But at that point [the time of the
Patriarchs], Torah had not yet been
given, yet it is written about Avraham,
'And he has kept my charge: [My
commandments, my laws, and my
teachings/Torah]' (Bereishit/Genesis
26:5). So from where did Avraham
learn the Torah?!
Rabbi Shimon says: his two kidneys
became like two pitchers of water, and
they flowed Torah.
And from where is it that this [is] so?
'My kidneys instruct me in morals at
night.[7]'"

וְעַד עַכְשָׁיו לֹא נִתְּנָה
תּוֹרָה, וּכְתִיב בְּאַבְרָהָם,
"וַיִּשְׁמֹר מִשְׁמַרְתִּי
[מִצְוֹתַי חֻקּוֹתַי וְתוֹרֹתָי]"
(בראשית כו:ה). וּמֵהֵיכָן
לִמַּד אברהם אֶת
הַתּוֹרָה?!
רבן שמעון אומר: נַעֲשׂוּ
שתי כליותיו כשתי כדים
של מים והיו נוֹבְעוֹת
תורה.
וּמִנַּיִן שכן הוא?
שנאמר, "אַף לֵילוֹת
יִסְּרוּנִי כִלְיוֹתָי" (תהלים
טז:ז).

Through donating a kidney, I have been able to understand
that Rabbi Shimon is not spinning a Patriarchs-as-Magicians
fairy tale, but is exposing a profound truth: Torah is the exter-
nalization of wisdom pulsating in potential in our bodies. Our
bodies are blueprints of Divine creation and wisdom and
like Torah, cannot survive without sharing of strength from
other bodies. Literally, everybody emerges into the world
from within another body: our existence is impossible without
profound bodily generosity and the sharing of organs. That I
was able to anticipate and make sense of some aspects of my
physical healing process on account of reflections shared with
me by several friends who have given birth via Caesarean

---

6. Bereishit Rabbah 95:3
7. Psalms 16:7

section further helped me locate my transplant in this frame of bodily interconnectedness.

Postscript

As expected, six weeks after transplant, I was given the green light to resume all physical activities. In the four weeks following, I danced for hours at two street festivals and a Phish concert, I swam numerous times in two lakes and one pool, went on two hikes, including one with strenuous rock scampering and maneuvering, and lifted big suitcases and other gear, all with no feelings of strain or discomfort in my abdominal area. (The dancing was a bit much for my 42-year-old knees, though!) Within the same summer, the recipient (at least the one I'm in touch with) remarked feeling vitality she hadn't felt in years. We have since shared many celebratory meals, Torah classes, and summer walks. Her life is remarkably full and lush. My scars are faint and I wear them as a badge of honor. I lost a body part I was barely using, and a little bit of time of full speed productivity. I gained beautiful new friends, strengthened other friendships, got to know my body better, learned a lot about human vulnerability and kindness, and, during those first two weeks, watched some solid TV shows I wouldn't have gotten around to seeing otherwise (Netflix's "The Get Down" will always have a warm spot in my heart).

May our bodies be vessels through which Torah flows and may our Torah reflect the wisdom in our bodies;

May our reception of Torah seamlessly involve sharing with others;

May we see our bodies as precious, shared inheritance[s] with all other bodies, all in need of mutual, tender care;

May we be like Avraham, learning Torah from our kidneys, so that our Torah works as a filter to help us retain all that is vital to us and to discharge that which is toxic;

May we approach life and Torah with the sensibility of abundance: just as we house abundant kidneys that can be shared, so should we house abundant Torah: with Torah and with everything we have, may we keep what we need and share our abundance with those who need it;

So that the words of our daily prayers ring true, that Torah's instructions are *"hayeinu v'orech yameinu,"* "our life and the length of our days."

Dr. Devora Steinmetz
The Torah of Chesed: Why I Became A Kidney Donor[8]

Last Sunday afternoon, I was wheeled into an operating room in Beilinson Hospital in Petach Tikva, an anesthesiologist said *laila tov* [good night], and a surgeon removed my left kidney, which was brought to an adjoining operating room and put into the abdomen of a twenty-three-year-old Israeli dental student from Georgia, FSU, whom I met for the first time three months ago.

I told very few people about my impending kidney donation before Sunday, mostly close family and friends, plus a few people with whom I had had to repeatedly cancel appointments in order to pursue the extensive regimen of medical tests, psychological testing, and [an] ethics committee interview that Israel has put in place in an attempt to ensure that donors are not offering their kidneys for personal gain, that they are not at unduly high risk for medical or psychological complications, and that they understand and have given sufficient consideration to their choice to become a living kidney donor. I have decided now to write publicly about my kidney donation in an attempt to call attention to the critical shortage of transplant

---

8. This was first published on May 22, 2012, in the *Jewish Week*, a New Jersey-based weekly newspaper.

organs – in Israel in particular – and to the opportunity to become a living kidney donor.

In addition, I want to explain my own choice to become a living donor and how I have come to understand my decision. This because I am all too aware that, while people openly tend to express admiration to the donor and to his or her family, there is all too often an assumption that a person who chooses to do such a thing is either a little crazy or exceptionally righteous – in either case, someone most unlike oneself and one's friends. Indeed, just last year, as I was in the process of testing for a different kidney patient (for whom I ended up not being a match), a mature and thoughtful student in my Talmud class used the example of "people who donate their kidney to a stranger" to illustrate the kind of person who is insufferably righteous – the kind of person of whom it's good to have a few in the world but whom you really don't want to be around.

The testing and interview process exacerbated this sense that I must be either crazy or a saint – "Please explain again why you want to donate a kidney." I explain[ed] why it makes sense to me. "Well, but most people don't make that decision, do they?" – Clearly, I was planning to do something that most people don't do, but the alternatives of seeing myself as a little crazy or as super-righteous both felt unacceptable – if there's one thing that seemed potentially worse than going through life thinking you're pretty weird, it's going through life thinking that you must be better than everyone else. So, I figured that I'd better shape a cogent way of seeing my choice that left both me and everyone around me looking both pretty sane and pretty good.

So, in line with the ethics committee's and psychologist's persistent questions, I want to explain first, why I chose to donate a kidney to a total stranger; and second, what I make of the fact that my decision is one that most people don't make.

The idea of donating a kidney first came to me when, twice over the course of several months, two of my children's day schools sent out a notice about a parent who needed a kidney, inquiring whether anyone in the community might consider being a donor. In both cases, a different donor was found, but in the process, I had begun to research the issue of organ shortages as well as the risks, short- and long-term, of being a living kidney donor. The situation seemed quite clear: there are simply not enough organs available from deceased donors to meet the needs of transplant patients, kidney donation surgery has proven to be very safe, and there don't seem to be any long-term health effects of living with only one kidney.

Donating a kidney seemed like a straightforward opportunity to save someone's life – an incredible privilege and an extraordinary mitzvah – and I decided that I would actively look for an opportunity to become a kidney donor. This meant, of course, that I would not be donating to a family member, something that most people seem to find quite reasonable, nor even most likely to someone in one of my extended communities, but rather to someone who would start out being a total stranger. I knew that, no matter how odd this act sometimes seemed even to me, if one of my children needed a kidney and no family member was a match, I would be actively searching for a potential donor, and I would be thrilled if a stranger would step forward to save my child. I couldn't see why the situation should look any different just because it was not my family who was in that devastating situation.

It had also come to my attention, during this learning process, that the issue of organ shortage is especially serious in Israel (for reasons that, it should be noted, go well beyond religious concerns). Until recently, a shockingly low percentage of Israelis had signed organ donation cards, ranking Israel at the very bottom of Western countries on organ donation.

(Happily, this has been changing due to a number of recent initiatives, including legislation encouraging people to sign up to be organ donors and a massive public awareness campaign explaining the issue of organ donation and offering people the opportunity to fill out organ donor cards.) Based on what I learned, I decided to try to donate a kidney in Israel. I began to see postings on a couple of Israeli community e-mail lists of which I'm a member about individuals who need a kidney, and that is how, ultimately, I found myself meeting the serious young student and his parents three months ago when we came to do cross-match testing at Beilinson.

He is not a family member, he is not a member of my community, his family could hardly be more different than my own. He was simply a person in need of someone to step forward and save his life, and I was a person who had the capacity to do that. The testing proved us to be a match. I was launched into months of testing and explaining, and last Sunday I gave him one of my kidneys.

So, what do I make of the fact that what seems so simple to me is something that most people would never think of doing?

Ten or so years ago in the Carlebach Shul, someone told me the following Torah [thought] that they had just learned from a friend: When someone does chesed for you, you want to find a way to pay them back, to reciprocate the chesed that they have done, but in most cases, you can't ever do that. Yet there is a way that you can pay them back, and that is by doing chesed for someone else. This teaching has stayed with me through some very difficult times. I have been the recipient of extraordinary chesed. Just around the time that I heard this Torah my family was dealing with a serious illness, and so many people helped us in ways that I could never have imagined and in ways that I knew I might never have done myself. And I knew that there was no way I could ever reciprocate. But what I could do was try to take opportunities that presented themselves to me to do *chesed* for others.

I am not scared by hospitals, I am not afraid of blood, I am not very sensitive to pain, and I'm a bit of a risk-taker. For me, donating a kidney was a rather easy thing to decide to do and to carry out. And it's something that's pretty clear-cut: the need is obvious, the way to help is obvious, the hoped-for result is clear. There are endless ways in which other people do *chesed* that I may be less good at – noticing the less-obvious pain or need of the person sitting near you, and reaching out to help him or her in small or large ways that may change their lives in ways that you might never know. The ways in which people helped our family might seem less dramatic or giving than the way in which I have helped the young man who now has my kidney, but I truly believe that they are equally heroic, and that just as these people might not be able to offer their kidneys, I might not be able to offer the kind of help that they did, or even notice that that kind of help is needed. I am not saying that I decided to donate a kidney in order to pay back the people who helped us. But I do believe that their acts of *chesed* enabled me to be more sensitive to the needs of others and to imagine extending myself in the way that I did to the young man who needed my help. This, I think, is the meaning of the Torah that I heard in the Carlebach Shul.

As I was preparing to leave Beilinson, my husband and I went to say goodbye to my kidney recipient and his parents. The young student and his father are shy, but the mother is effusive. She wants to buy me things, to send me presents, to send my family on a vacation to the Dead Sea. I have told her over and over that I don't want anything, that I can't take anything, but she persists. So finally, I told her the Torah that I'd heard in the Carlebach Shul, and I blessed her son and her and her husband with many years of good health full of many opportunities to do *chesed* for others. And then something incredible happened. This woman who had been trying to shower me with boxes of chocolate and perfume told me that she and her son had discussed a plan for when he finishes school and becomes a dentist – that he would set aside one day each month, in my name, to treat people who can't afford to pay. I don't know whether he will do exactly that, but I did feel, in a most powerful way, that this young man and his parents were now recipients of the Torah that I had learned, the Torah of *chesed*, and that my own act, like the acts of those who have done *chesed* for me and my family, will generate more acts of *chesed* in the world.

Each of us has the capacity to do tremendous acts of *chesed*. And each of us has different ways in which we are capable of doing *chesed*. Donating a kidney is one way that made sense for me. If you think it might make sense for you, please feel free to contact me (desteinmetz@gmail.com), and I can help you find the information that you need to make your decision or put you in touch with someone who can help match you with someone whose life you can save. If this is not your path of *chesed*, then know that you have ways to help someone else that may be just as powerful and life-saving. As we approach the festival of the giving of our beautiful Torah,[9] may we all be privileged to find our own path in the Torah of *chesed*.

Aaron Nielsenschultz

I met the man to whom I would end up donating a kidney on Wednesday, October 12, 2016. I remember the date not because our meeting was auspicious, which it wasn't – it was a brief

---

9. This article was written shortly before the holiday of Shavuot, on which the receiving of the Torah is celebrated.

introduction in passing, a wish for an easy fast. Neither of us knew the other or the other's story at that point. No, I remember the date so easily because it was Yom Kippur, and months later, when I reflected on my journey to donating a kidney, the realization that we had met on that day left me speechless.

But for me, the journey to being a living kidney donor began a full two years before I met my recipient. In June 2015, I learned that my friend and teacher, Rabbi Dr. Shmuly Yanklowitz, donated one of his kidneys in an act of altruism. Having learned with and worked with Rav Shmuly, I was not surprised that he would undertake such a selfless gesture, and I was happy to read about his thought process, his progress to surgery, and his amazing recovery after the fact. "How wonderful," I remember thinking, and wondered, "Would I ever be willing to do such a thing?" It was an abstraction, this thought – one I did not imagine would be on my mind anytime soon.

I didn't think too much more about the question until I received an email from my congregation, where I serve as Director of Religious School, in November of 2016, relating that one of our members was in end–stage kidney failure and that he needed a kidney. I did not realize yet that M.S., the man who needed the kidney, was the man I had met on Yom Kippur a month before. Instead, that abstract question from more than two years before echoed back into my brain, and for the first time I looked at it as a concrete proposition rather than an abstraction.

With Rav Shmuly as an inspiration, I first spent some time researching the medical side of kidney donation. The numbers are shocking: over 100,000 people are waiting in the United States for a kidney transplant, and only about 17,000 transplants are done per year. More than two thirds of these are cadaver transplants, with living kidney donations making up only somewhat more than 5,000 donations. This [is so] despite the fact that so many of us carry an extra kidney our whole lives; our two kidneys perform four times the amount of filtration our bodies need.

Within no time, I resolved that I would enter the testing phase to see if I could match with M.S., and were that not to work out, I would sign up for an undirected donation. I did not need both of my kidneys, and so I would surely find someone who could use my spare.

Naturally, I spoke about the idea of donation with my wife and children; my wife had worked as a critical care nurse and understood the risks and benefits better than anyone, and my children reported being wholly unsurprised that I would be willing to do such a thing. I spoke with our senior rabbi – who serves as both my rabbi as well as my immediate supervisor – and we spent a fair amount of time hashing out possibilities and alternatives before he gave me his personal and professional blessing.

The process to become a kidney donor offered me a unique glimpse into the healthcare world. I have always been a healthy person, and the variety of tests, exams, and procedures that I endured on my way to becoming a kidney donor all had one goal in mind: determining just how healthy I was. How different a feeling this process created in me, I imagined, as compared to so many of the others I met in waiting rooms: those with fearful diagnoses to be borne out, or those facing arduous paths to recovery, or those confronting the prospect that recovery would not come. For me, each test confirmed my health and suitability. In no time, M.S. and I were both cleared for surgery.

The surgery went off without a hitch, and within twenty-four hours I was able to walk to M.S.'s room to visit with him; I could see the color returning to his face, and more than that, I could see the life returning to him – and not just to him but also to his wife and children, to his father. I was humbled by their gratitude; by giving one kidney, I had brought joy and positivity, hope for a future to all of them. They [now] had time together, and the fear of losing their father, husband, son no longer gripped them the same way. The words of Yosef Yitzchak Schneersohn – the Frierdiker Rebbe[10] – came to me: "Time must be guarded... Every bit of time, every day that passes, is not just a day but a life's concern." I had thought I was donating a kidney, but I came to realize that M.S. received time, renewed purpose – life itself.

M.S. likes to say that it was a miracle we met. For me, I think the whole process underlined something the sages in the Talmud teach us in Tractate *Ta'anit*: that we should not count on miracles.[11] Instead, we have to count on each other, on our fellow people – we need to count on our teachers to inspire us, count on our families and communities to support us, and even count on strangers to save us. Another dear friend and teacher of mine, Rabbi Mark Levin, says, "We are the community we need." Sometimes we don't see it; sometimes we downplay our own role in building and fostering that community.

And sometimes it takes the sanctity of Yom Kippur to remind us that holiness can be ours every day.

---

10. The Frierdeker Rebbe was the sixth rebbe (grand rabbi) of the Lubavitch sect of Hasidism.
11. Babylonian Talmud, Ta'anit 9a

Chapter 8
Interviews

Professor Peter Singer[1]

RABBI DR. SHMULY YANKLOWITZ: Professor Peter Singer, thank you for talking with me. I've been teaching your ideas for a long time and it's really an honor to talk with you about the topic of organ donation. What do you think is the best moral and philosophical argument for living organ donation? Is it a moral obligation or merely a kind gesture of altruism?

PROFESSOR PETER SINGER: The best argument for [living organ donation] is that there are people who, because of kidney disease or living on dialysis, have a quality of life that is poor and whose life expectancy is significantly reduced. On the other hand, healthy people with two kidneys can do well with one kidney; we don't really need two kidneys. The chances that you will suffer greatly or even have a shorter life because of donating a kidney are really small. One estimate I've seen is one in four thousand and it may

---

1. Professor Peter Singer is a utilitarian philosopher, the child of parents who fled the Holocaust. He teaches at Princeton University and at the University of Melbourne.

even be less than that if you are not suffering from various other medical conditions. Therefore, you can do a lot more good – your kidney can do a lot more good – in someone else's body than in your own.

Now does that mean it's a moral obligation? That's tough. In one sense, from the utilitarian point of view (which I think is the correct ethical point of view), yes, we really ought to do what will have the best consequences, and donating a kidney *will* have the best consequences. But to use a heavy term like saying it's your 'moral obligation' may be counterproductive in a way. It might make people feel terribly guilty if they *don't* do it. And because there are few people doing it at the moment – there are some and it's growing, but it's still a tiny proportion of the eligible population as a whole – I think the language may be a bit too heavy for that. Some might think that somehow you're doing something really badly wrong if you don't donate a kidney, whereas in fact you're not doing the right thing perhaps, but you're doing what most people are doing – that is, not donating a kidney to people who need it. I'd rather praise people who do donate [than] condemn or blame people who don't donate.

YANKLOWITZ: Do you believe having a second kidney could be viewed as a luxury? And how does your argument about the moral problem regarding buying coffee as opposed to donating money for a malaria net apply to this scenario? Is an organ fundamentally different from one's money or is it another form of luxury that can be comparable?

SINGER: There's something slightly funny about saying that something that you're born with and that everybody else has is a luxury. I suppose you could say, "Well why did we evolve to have two kidneys?" I don't know the answer to that. Maybe it's about symmetry?

One couldn't have called it a luxury until we had the ability to remove one and save someone's life or greatly benefit somebody from it. But that's only recently. I suppose you could say that the development of medical technology for transplanting a kidney has made having two kidneys something that is optional because we don't really need two. So yes, in that strict sense of the term, it's a *luxury*. Now, you asked how does it compare with the luxuries of going out and buying a coffee or buying bottled water when the water that comes out of your tap is safe to drink. Those things are luxuries too. The answer to that is that it's a lot easier to *not* buy the bottled water and, unless you're a real coffee addict, to just pass up the coffee or to make the coffee at home where you save a couple of dollars by doing that. That's a lot easier for most people than going into a hospital, having a kidney removed and taking a few days off work. And people do worry about the idea that something may go wrong. I know I said that the chances are small, but it's possible. So that's the difference: that one of them is easy to do and there's, in a way, no excuse for not doing it. The other one, I can empathize more with people who feel that this is a much bigger deal.

YANKLOWITZ: Moving from personal choice to societal incentives, do you believe we should open up the market for selling organs? Of course, the concern there has always been about exploitation of the poor. On the other hand, if a model could be put in place where no one [would] be on dialysis and no one would die of renal failure, would it be worth it?

SINGER: Yes, but I don't think we should have an unregulated market. We need a different model than that. Because not only could it lead to exploitation of the poor, but it could also mean that only the rich can get these organs. And I don't really think that how rich one is ought to be critical to whether you live or die; unfortunately, that is often how it is. I'd like to reduce that to the greatest extent I can, so what I imagine is a regulated system.

And that system provides incentives for people to donate an organ. I would use the word *donate* rather than *sell*, because I would be thinking of incentives that provide lasting benefits. Rather than a cash payment – which as you can imagine, people might spend on getting drugs or they might gamble or whatever it might be, and then they're worse off, I'm thinking of things like providing them with long-term income, some sort of fund that pays them a dividend on a regular basis, or education for their children (if they have children). Clearly health insurance – long-term health insurance – that they don't have to pay for would be a valuable thing. I think we could provide some long-term incentives that would mean they would not be exploited and they would not end up in a private transaction where some wealthy person says, "Hey, I'll pay you one hundred thousand dollars for your kidney." Rather, the kidneys would be allocated by hospitals to the next person on the waiting list independently of that person's means.

YANKLOWITZ: Do you think our policies around end-of-life decisions should be different, given the amount of expenses that go towards maintaining people on end-of-life care and given the number of lives we could save through end-of-life organ donation?

SINGER: Certainly, I think our policy should be different. Depending on what part of the United States you're in – because a number of states including all of the West Coast and (I think) Vermont and a couple of others – do now allow people to have the assistance of a physician in ending their life. And that clearly gives people something that they want as well as reducing medical expenses. Incidentally, I don't think that reducing medical expenses should ever be the primary reason for someone to choose to end their life. But it's really crazy to keep people alive at great expense in the hospital when they themselves rationally decide that they don't want to go on living, that their quality of life is too poor, [when] they have no prospect of recovery from the condition that they're dying from. So, I favor legislation allowing people to choose to have physician assistance in dying.

And when that happens of course, people could elect to donate their organs. Certainly, at that point, it's a much easier thing to do; you have no further use for them. You don't have to worry about something going wrong. I think everybody, at the end of life, should think about what organs they are capable of donating.

YANKLOWITZ: One of the main reasons that some people share with me why they don't want to donate a kidney is lest a family member might need an organ in the future. How might or might not utilitarian thought show familial preference? That one might save their kidney for a potential family member rather than give immediately to a stranger?

SINGER: I understand that. I think utilitarian thinking just has to accept that we are mammals, which means we care about our close relatives. That's obviously necessary for our genes to survive: that we look after our children – that we don't just look after them, but that we love them and think about them. And there is a close link between our happiness and the happiness of our children and other close family members. We have to accept this. It's not something we're going to change or indeed something that we really should change. I think what we need to do is to think of a model for overcoming that. And one would be to say that anybody who does donate a kidney gets priority for kidneys that will become available should they be needed, not only for themselves but also for their immediate family members. (You would have to define [family members]: Obviously their children, or maybe their siblings, or something like that.) You would give them a guarantee that if this were to happen, which is unlikely but it will happen occasionally, that those they love would be looked after in that situation.

YANKLOWITZ: My last question is a quick one: Have people told you that your arguments have ever led them to donate a kidney?

SINGER: Yes, I have heard that from a couple of people actually. A guy named Chris Croy wrote to me and said that my argument about donating to save the lives of people in extreme poverty (for example, by giving to some of the organizations recommended on www.thelifeyoucansave .org) was discussed in his class, [and that] this led him to donate his kidney. Chris said that after thinking about this question for a while, he was led to approach a hospital to donate a kidney and he did so, and he's happy that he's done that. So, I've heard from a couple who were influenced. I find it impressive that the power of philosophical argument is so great that somebody will do that.

The Many Dimensions of Kidney Donation: An Interview with Dr. John Fung

RABBI DR. SHMULY YANKLOWITZ: With more than thirty years of experience, Dr. John Fung is a renowned leader in the field of organ transplantation including liver, kidney, pancreas, islet, and intestinal transplantation. Dr. Fung's dedication to innovation and delivering the highest level of patient care is recognized through his consistent appearance on America's top doctors and best doctors in America list.

He serves as a professor and the director of transplant surgery at the University of Chicago.

YANKLOWITZ: Dr. Fung, thank you for taking the time to talk.

DR. JOHN FUNG: Pleasure, Rabbi.

YANKLOWITZ: I have long admired you and your work, so it really means a great deal for you to take this time to talk with me. Do you believe that more people should be thinking about and considering altruistic living kidney donation?

FUNG: Yes, I think kidney donation from a live donor is one of the oldest forms of donation. It was the source of organs for kidney transplantation before brain death, so the first transplants that were successful were from living donors. I think the concept of altruistic, undirected donation, in other words, from somebody who just wants to donate to an anonymous recipient on the kidney waiting list is really somewhat new. Over the past five to seven years, live organ donation has been popularized through mechanisms that allow better matching to occur in a more objective way and in a way that is more transparent, not only to the recipient, but to the donor and to the general public. So, altruistic living donation is truly a way to increase the organ donor pool, particularly in the way that we deal with these multiple chains. It's important in helping to facilitate matching in ways that we had never done before.
I think it's a noble effort.

YANKLOWITZ: How would you say that some of these trends have changed in living kidney donation? You already started touching on it. Also, what do you expect to see in the next ten years? Any possible new trends?

FUNG: Clearly, the idea of swapping as we call it – which means that you find incompatible pairs where they don't match – is a positive trend. Say you have couple one and couple two, and somehow couple two, which is also not compatible with each other, are now compatible with the other couple. So that's a simple concept of a swap. Eventually, this led to better matching, better not only for tissue typing, but for patients who may be what we call "sensitized" (which means that they have antibodies against the donor). This allows for able-matching, and it increases the opportunity for people to be living donors, and to facilitate, as I mentioned, these swaps and chains.

Going forward, I think we also have a better understanding of the risks for a living donor. There are some risks, although small, but I think we're much better able to understand the biology. For example, some African-Americans have a gene that makes them more likely to develop kidney disease later in life. If we can identify these risk factors, then we may be able to protect the donor rate even more. I think going forward also in the area of desensitization and finding mechanisms to further enhance the opportunity for highly sensitized patients for kidney transplantation is down the road. And then finally, looking maybe ten or twenty years down the line, things like bio-artificial kidneys and transplants from genetically modified animals...Clearly those are kind of way out there, but if we're trying to see what's going on, what we currently do now with our source of cadaveric donors and living donors, I think we are making some advances [in that direction]. But we still have 80,000 people waiting for a kidney here in the United States, and so we've got a long way to go.

YANKLOWITZ: Do I understand that we're moving in a direction where even if there's not a match or not strong compatibility, that there's still a way to make a transplant possible?

FUNG: Yes. When you look at the chance that two individuals will be matched so that their transplant outcomes are going to be better, it is really hit and miss. So randomly, if you were to look at the opportunity for two non-related individuals to be matched identically, it's probably on the order of about one in a million. Now, you don't have to get into that level of matching in order for a kidney transplant to be successful. Certainly, we have much lower degrees of matching that have been successful. But there are individuals, particularly women and people who've had a failed kidney transplant before, who've become sensitized: they've had a previous blood transfusion or whatever, and it makes it more difficult to find a matched kidney.

So, the idea of being able to get the largest donor pool available to find the right matching to avoid some of the worst kinds of situations where there's an antibody against the donor – those are the situations where, as I mentioned, these kinds of swaps, these computer-generated algorithms – looking at large donor lists of volunteers, living donors, and cadaveric donors – gives the opportunity for these highly sensitized patients to get a kidney. That's really the only way to do it, to do it in a cost effective and, I think, a predictably successful way.

YANKLOWITZ: What are some of the possible paths that we could take in the coming decades to end the need to donate organs at all?

FUNG: Clearly, the best way to avoid the need to deal with a growing list of patients on the waiting list is to deal with finding ways to reduce incidents of kidney disease. We know the risk factors for kidney disease include hypertension (particularly in the African-American population), high blood pressure, which, when uncontrolled, leads to increased stress on the kidneys and, ultimately, kidney failure. Certain drugs, like excessive use of non-steroidal, anti-inflammatory agents like Ibuprofen, can also increase the risk for kidney damage. Diabetes, which is a growing problem in our increasingly larger American population, is also a risk factor.

And then there are genetic factors. Those are things that we can start to focus on which can help prevent kidney disease. I think this is the best way, because of the eighty thousand people who are on the kidney waiting list, there are probably ten times that number of people who actually have chronic kidney disease or are not eligible for a kidney transplant because of other factors. So, clearly, we have to reduce the incidence of end–stage kidney disease first.

YANKLOWITZ: Zooming out to the political and global level, what do you think about the ethical question of opening up a regulated marketplace for kidney sales for transplants?

FUNG: This is a good question, Rabbi. There are two camps globally: those that have advocated that we should explore incentivized donation, and the bulk of the community which has resisted it. I can say that, probably, the bulk of the transplant community's leaders are against regulated, incentivized donation, but clearly there are incentives that are perhaps not as tangible [as money]. These can be things like providing prolonged health care insurance for donors and other benefits that may not be equivalent to cash.

Societies that have had incentivized organ donation have found that there have been ethical dilemmas that are generated: if you think about that kind of market, you're going to have a population that is wealthy, that is going to take advantage of the situation, and those that are less economically fortunate who are going to be the ones brokering their kidneys for these incentives. While I think you could conceptually come up with a system – which on the surface looks not as commercialized as you might want it to be – the problem is that these systems tend to become unregulated; other breaches and ethics come into play.

So just in general, I think there are a lot of challenges to have organ sales or incentivized organ donation. At least at this point, we have not really exhausted all the opportunities that we have for both deceased donation as well as living donation.

YANKLOWITZ: Is the thinking in the transplant community – where the bulk of opposition is coming from – that the exploitation of the donor matters more than the potential to save life? Is that rooted in an ethic that "do no harm" is principle number one?

FUNG: Yes, I think that's exactly the way they're saying it, particularly with regard to living donation. Donor safety is the primal and primary driving thought when it comes to organ donation and transplantation. In the deceased donor situation, which makes up the bulk of the transplants in the United States, particularly for lifesaving organs like heart, liver, [and] lungs, that issue is not as germane because the organ donors are deceased. But we still have issues that we want to tackle in terms of making sure that the donor's wishes are carried out, and that the family's wishes are also respected to an extent where [donating] doesn't negate the organ donor's original desire.

But when it comes to living donors, the primal directive is: do no harm.

YANKLOWITZ: There are many opportunities, obviously, for cadaveric donation. Can you briefly walk us through other living donation opportunities? Which organs are we talking about, and whether or not, and to what extent, you recommend those?

FUNG: Kidney donation makes up 99% of living donation when it comes to donated organs, at least in the United States. In parts of the world, where deceased donor efforts are not as robust as in the West, particularly in Asia, then living donors of kidneys are truly welcome. While it's still number one, the second most common type of transplants are living donors for liver transplants: since you can take a liver and partition it in certain ways, the liver will regenerate to some extent, [and] you can do living [donation] of a partial liver graft for transplantation, particularly from adults to children. This has been practiced now for about twenty years. More recently, [donating] larger pieces of liver from the donor into an adult recipient, which is a little bit more challenging, and has a little bit more risk, [is being performed as well].

So, in general, the risk for a living liver donor compared to a living kidney donor is probably about a one in two hundred risk of dying in a living liver donor versus a kidney donor, which itself is about one in two to three thousand; so, there is a risk for both, but the risk is a one-fold magnitude greater for a liver donor than for a kidney donor.

YANKLOWITZ: What about lung transplants?

FUNG: That's really fallen out of favor. There have been living donor lung transplants that have been done in the past. Generally, the amount of lung that you can remove from a donor is insufficient for one recipient. You may actually have to have two donors for one recipient which means you have the potential for 300% or more mortality. Lungs in the United States and most parts of the world are not optimally utilized: there are many more lungs that are being discarded than there are being transplanted.

YANKLOWITZ: So, my last two questions are relevant to the Jewish conversation on cadaveric donation. The first is when one decides if they want to donate organs – after the cessation of a heartbeat, defining death then, or at the death of the brainstem. Of course, with cessation of heartbeat there won't be much left but with brainstem death one of the concerns is how will brain death be diagnosed? What is the medical standard today in terms of defining brain death?

FUNG: So, brain death means there is no blood flow to the brain. And that means that there is no possibility for that person to be weaned off of the ventilator or life support with any chance of physiologic function. In other words, once you remove the ventilator, there is no way that the patient – that person, that donor – is going to breathe on their own; they will eventually die. Without the endocrine component of it, your body will slowly wither away.

So, if the brain stem is alive, it still has blood, but that donor – that body – would have no cognitive function – but it could still potentially breathe on its own; that's not brain death. When we do the cranial reflexes and when we do these blood flow studies of the brain, that's not equal to brain death. When we talk about brain death, all of those functions are gone.

YANKLOWITZ: Obviously, you can't return from brain death. So, when these stories pop up in the news every day of someone returning from brain death, does that just mean it was misdiagnosed?

FUNG: Absolutely. To be stringent about declaring brain death, you have met the criteria. In other words, the donor or the person being evaluated cannot have had any type of sedative in the past twenty-four hours, they can't have any detectable levels of brain activity, they have to be warmed to normal body temperature (because hypothermia can sometimes also suppress brain function). Then, it takes neurologic exams and or radiological exams within a given period of time, usually 24 hours apart (with or without EEG-monitoring), to define brain death.

If you read these stories, it could be because that person was, for example, hypothermic and had no reflexes when they were cold but then when the body warmed up and the blood was circulating, blood was getting back to the brain, then that donor's neurologic functions could return to some extent. These kinds of stories that you read about, there's always a lack of understanding of what the situation was that caused that misdiagnosis to occur.

YANKLOWITZ: Jewish law has been strongly in favor of donating to directly save life, and the question of donating one's body to medical research has, in some limited cases in Jewish law, been permitted, when the body afterwards could be buried. This comes up in Israel, but in America is there a possibility in the medical research world of a body being buried after [being donated for medical research] or is the body, by rule, always discarded?

FUNG: For example, we don't do this much in the anatomy labs where you have bodies donated for dissection and teaching, but those bodies for research or teaching in any academic institution are treated as if they're recently deceased and you plan to bury, donate, cremate or do otherwise. All of the components that are part of the research activities are treated as if they are your loved one. There is a lot of respect paid to bodies that are donated for research. I can tell you; we do a ceremony every year in the medical school that recognizes those generous donations that allow us to do our research and teaching. I don't know the details about the bodies that are requested to be buried in a grave, how they actually transfer that…

YANKLOWITZ: But somebody could make that request?

FUNG: Yes, they could.

YANKLOWITZ: Dr. Fung, thank you so much for your time. You are doing the most amazing work in the world. I am a huge fan.

FUNG: Thank you, Rabbi Shmuly. I have to admit, that I'm really impressed with your support of organ donation and your own personal travels through that donation process are impressive. Good luck.

YANKLOWITZ: Thank you.

An Interview with Judy Firestone Singer, from Matnat Chayim

RABBI DR. SHMULY YANKLOWITZ: To start off, can you just tell us what Matnat Chayim does?

JUDY FIRESTONE SINGER: Matnat Chayim is an Israeli non-profit which recruits and supports healthy volunteers who want to donate a kidney to people who need transplants.

YANKLOWITZ: Wonderful. I've heard that the numbers for your organization are up to 500 now?

SINGER: Yes, in a couple of days [January 2018], we will have our five hundredth transplant. And the vast majority of our donors do not know their recipients. All of them do it on a completely voluntary basis. And it's an amazing privilege to be able to take part.

YANKLOWITZ: Israelis have traditionally had a low rate of organ donations. Why is that?

SINGER: Partly, I think it's on religious grounds. There are debates among the Orthodox and ultra-Orthodox communities about time of death – cardiac death versus brain death – and that prevents many Orthodox and ultra-Orthodox Jews... they feel that they cannot donate after their death. Also, I think a lot of it is just cultural and even superstition. People who feel like, "Well you know, when the Messiah comes, I want to have all my parts, so I don't miss out on all the excitement." It's not something that's logical. It's an emotional sort of antipathy to the idea of donating; and Israel didn't have huge success in getting organ donors to sign organ donor cards, relative to other countries.

YANKLOWITZ: How has this started the change in recent years?

SINGER: Two main things happened: First, in 2008, the Knesset passed the Transplant Law which, on the one hand, stopped Israelis from going abroad to various third world and other countries to get transplants, many of which were not done in the most legal and moral manner. The same law also gave certain incentives to people to do living donations. People are now compensated for lost work days, transportation, health insurance, and various other things. These provisions allow people to become living organ donors without losing money. That's thing number one that happened.

Around the same time in 2009, Matnat Chayim was founded, and the organization actively recruited healthy volunteers to donate organs. And it's become a real success story. It's even a trend in Israel: people who have friends who have donated, they get interested; people who see one of our organization's publications or see something on the news; or it goes from word of mouth. Many people in Israel now know somebody who has donated a kidney. Israel is a family-based society and everybody knows everybody. And the more people who know someone who has donated, the more likely they are to get interested and start researching it themselves.

YANKLOWITZ: What are some of the main incentives that Israel offers for living organ donation? Are these incentives helping?

SINGER: It's not so much that the donations are caused by these incentives. It's just [that] when a person has decided they want to do this amazing *mitzvah*, this amazing good deed, they will not suffer any financial hardship because their salary will be paid, the transportation costs will be paid... This a big thing in the States: people flying back and forth and such. There isn't always someone who will pay the expenses, and there's never someone who will pay their lost wages. That's a big thing. Not everybody can afford to take a month off of work to help somebody else out.

So, the financial incentives will cover any losses that people may have. People get their life insurance paid for five years, they get their health insurance paid for five years, which is a great thing. And also, both for signing a donor card and for donating an organ and being a living donor, the donor and their entire immediate family – parents, children, and siblings – all get bumped up on the list if they themselves ever need an organ. So, if any of my kids, God forbid, ever need a kidney or a heart or a liver, they will automatically go to the head of the line because of my donation.

That's a big deal, because many times when someone is considering donating a kidney, people say to them, "What if one of your own kids needs one someday?" This legislation, which is enlightened and unique, has taken away a lot of the apprehension that people feel about organ donation. I think it's one of the big reasons why Israel is now the country which has the highest rate of altruistic kidney donation in the world. I really think that our organization and this legislation are models for other countries and other communities as they try to understand how to help kidney patients and people on dialysis.

YANKLOWTZ: I'm blown away by the work you do. It's incredibly inspiring to me to learn more about the work of Matnat Chayim. Thank you so much.

SINGER: Thank you.

Chapter 9
A Recipient's Story

An Article by Yossi (the recipient of my kidney) Written Shortly After the Transplant

You need courage to live, so it's important to me that you read this. Please give me a few minutes of your time and let this story accompany you for a while. I know that it doesn't have to do with you. Maybe it doesn't concern you. Or maybe it touches you for just a moment; it might even be moving. But then it just fades away. It is extremely important to me that my story stays with everyone so that, maybe, there will be a chance for more people to save themselves and start their new life.

It's not easy for me to tell this story – my personal story – with which I have been dealing for years; I'm a private person. But ever since I have been through it, I have decided that it is crucial that I raise awareness on the subject. That I had reached rock bottom, and that I need to help more people and friends that were in the same bad situation as me. And I feel that something inside of me is encouraging me to act.

I always wanted to be an actor. I even went to acting school for years. I used to fantasize about it, I wanted it so bad. I still do. But instead of acting on a stage in the theater, I got to act on a stage much more meaningful: The stage of life.

When I was sixteen years old, I was diagnosed with renal

failure. I managed to withhold this information until I was 29. After I turned 29, I got worse and fast. A few months after my birthday, I began dialysis; my life was on hold. Apart from my family, no one really knew about my situation. Life froze for an unknown period of time. I hadn't done anything and it was horrible. Two years went by with harsh, exhausting treatments: three times a week, four hours each time. And at the most depressing place: a hospital.

It's important to understand that dialysis is only a temporary solution. It's important to understand that after a few years without a kidney transplant, the dialysis wears out the body which can lead to death. People kept asking me what exactly I had on my arm. It was a fistula, a developed vein that is stabbed during every treatment with big, wide needles. Through them, the blood leaves the body into the dialysis machine and into a strainer that is essentially an artificial device that replaces natural kidney function.

There are two options for a person experiencing renal failure: One is to go through a kidney transplant from a person – dead or alive. So, first of all I would like to encourage each and every one of you out there to sign an organ donation card (EDI in Israel). It is vital for you do so. The other action you can do is donate a kidney.

Yes, I am well aware that it sounds scary and larger than life. And that is a part of the problem: people are either unaware of the process or they really don't know much about it. Today, the procedure is simple, and you are discharged after just two days, back to your regular, normal life.

The day after going through a transplant, I can honestly say that I have a new life. My life is *mine* again. I want to see this chance at a new life belong to more men, women, children, teenagers, young adults and grown-ups that I have seen and known throughout these years. Unfortunately, some are no longer with us. Those who are, survive, but they continue waiting in a long line, years of waiting as things get worse. (If you are wondering about my donor...he's doing great! He is back to his good old life. He gained a new brother in the process and a great deal of satisfaction that he had been fortunate to save someone's life.)

It can't be easy thinking about the possibly of donating a kidney to someone you don't know, just as much as if you *do* know them. I assure you that it is not easy to ask someone for a donation, even *if* that someone is family.

It isn't a simple prospect to consider, but if you explore and listen to stories of people who have done so, those who had the greatest joy there is, of saving someone's life, they will tell you it has been their privilege to donate and to save that individual, that it has given them the most significant kind of joy there is in this world.

As far as I'm concerned, every person who donates a kidney is a superhero. Every one of those people is an individual with a strong sense of will, great power, and a lot of love; they are not selfish. They think of ways to help another. They come from an inner place of love and the belief that they can do something – anything – to save someone else's life.

About a year ago, I came to New York to try my luck. *Maybe here I have a better chance to receive a kidney and not waste my life on dialysis.* And, exactly a year later, just as I was going through a dialysis treatment, I received the fateful phone call. It was the happiest phone call of my life, that there was a donor that had heard my story and was so moved by it that he decided that he wanted to save my life.

A person from the other side of the world saved me! Can you believe it?!

If people were aware of the situation, more people would be saved every year from preventable death.

The man who saved my life, his name is Shmuly, a rabbi, married with kids. He lives in Arizona and is an educator. I didn't know much about him until that emotional meeting on the day of my surgery. It was very early in the morning. I was excited when the doors opened and I saw him.

I couldn't speak.

All I could do was cry out loud.

I was overwhelmed. When something like this happens, you don't really know what to feel. How do you prepare yourself for such a meeting? All we could do is hold each other and cry. Together. After a short conversation, I could tell that this is an amazing, sensitive person, one who was more worried about me than he was about himself. I had the same feeling as he did: I was worried about him much more than I was about me.

A few minutes later, they took Shmuly to the operating room while I was being prepped for surgery. The transplant passed. So did the pain. All that was left was a strong sensation of the human strength to do things that are larger than life. The joy I felt for having my life back and the joy he felt for saving one's life is something that I can't even put into words.

After the pain had passed, I slowly began to realize that I *finally* had a functioning kidney. It's said that you only live once, but I felt like I got a chance to live life for a second time. I waited for this moment for so long and I know now that I had a crazy experience, filled with emotions that I've never felt before. Suddenly, you understand and see life from a whole different angle, a deeper one, a powerful one. Suddenly, you understand the power of life, the power of helping one another; the forces that exist in this world.

I've heard doctors say: "We were born with two kidneys: one to live with and one to donate and save life with." We have no need for two kidneys. One kidney can do the exact same job that two kidneys do together. Anyone who has received a kidney in a transplant, a kidney that previously did not belong to him, lives years with it. They live a normal life, just as the one who had donated the kidney.

I say: What is crazier, more exciting, and powerful than the fact that not only did God give us life, but He gave us the privilege to give life to another!

To all of you who've read this and were touched by my story, I say: Please, *do something* about it. Remember that the will to live is just as powerful as the will to save. Remember that God gave us not only life, but the chance to give life to other people. To all of you who've read this, I thank you. And if you're not tired yet and would like to keep going, I do have few more things to say.

After the transplant, I stayed with an amazing couple that I had met just as I started the treatments: Carmit and Shmuli. Shmuli donated his kidney to Carmit several years before and, ever since, they decided that they wished to take part in the process of those who needed to have a transplant. I am fortunate and happy that it was me.

Carmit accompanied me through it all. She did not leave my side from the moment I arrived in New York, even when I was still in Israel. Before my flight to America, she was there on an everyday basis to calm, support, and encourage me. Just as she was there for me, so was her family. Shmuli was there to help and to calm me before and after the transplant. Thanks to them, the entire process was so much easier. I can honestly write that I have the privilege to know them and thank them over and over again for everything. It isn't an obvious thing to do. I can't thank them enough.

I want to thank all the wonderful people doing divine service. Jewish individuals that don't care who you are or what you are; they're just there to help. They spend every day, every minute recruiting and bringing together donors and the ones who need them. They devote their lives and accompany everyone through the whole process. They support, visit and they become close friends. Thank you to Renewal.

I couldn't have done this without my sister. It wouldn't have been the same. She's been there from the start of the dialysis, throughout the transplant and to this day. She didn't leave my side. For this, I want to thank you, Ronit.

Last, but not least, I want to thank the one who saved my life, my brother Shmuly. *Thank you* does not even begin to cover all that I want to say for what you did for me. And if there was a greater word to say, I would have said it by now. I wish for you and your wife and children much happiness in life, a lot of joy and light, health and strength, faith and love. I wish more people would do what you have done for me: save lives. God gives us life, but He also gives us the privilege and possibility to give life to each other. And *you* were a part of it.

Thank you.[1]

---

1. Many thanks to Inbal Donenfeld for translating this essay into English from the original Hebrew.

Chapter 10

About Organizations in the Field

Renewal

Renewal: Bringing Hope to Those Who Need It Most

For those with chronic kidney disease, the process of receiving a new kidney from a live donor (or even a deceased donor) is daunting and difficult to navigate. Renewal, a nonprofit based in Brooklyn, New York, provides guidance and counseling for potential donors, as well as support for those who suffer from kidney failure. The organization educates and creates awareness about live kidney donation so that potential donors will consider helping those in need, and then accompanies both the donor and the recipient through the entire procedure. Renewal is there every step of the way, making sure everyone feels supported and has everything they need. In addition, Renewal strives to cover as many of the extraneous expenses as possible that the donor might have, such as travel fares, lodging, and even lost wages.

I've been touched personally by the kindness that Renewal shows to the Jewish community and the world. When I underwent my kidney donation journey, I reached out to the staff of Renewal and they guided me the whole way through. I had so many questions and concerns before my procedure; everything felt overwhelming. Thankfully, Renewal assisted me with my due diligence from my first questions until my convalescence. It is this personal touch that makes Renewal such a special and unique Jewish organization. Renewal wants to make the process of donation as easy and (relatively) painless as possible, so that more people within the Jewish community will consider becoming living organ donors. For that reason, a Renewal staff member works closely with each donor throughout the entire process, attending appointments and evaluations, as well as accompanying the donor on the day of their surgery.

Without Renewal, I wouldn't have had an institutional partner to carry me through the many steps of the organ donation process.

If your curiosity has been piqued, Renewal's website is filled with information about kidney disease and live donation, in the form of articles, testimonies, and videos.[1] The FAQs page of the website discusses the benefits of living donation, stating that, on average, live kidneys last twice as long as "deceased" kidneys. The page also states that the majority of people waiting for a transplant – a wait which usually lasts several years – will not make it past five years on dialysis. As the website makes clear, that is why it is even more important for Renewal to match donors and recipients as quickly as possible. In a truly moving testimonial, a grateful recipient recounts that if it hadn't been for Renewal pairing him with a donor within a year of being put on the transplant list, he likely would have had to wait upwards of six years for a kidney, and probably would have died. Had it not been for Renewal, a beautiful soul would have been lost.

---

1. Learn more at www.renewal.org.

Renewal saves lives while also upholding the purest essence of Jewish ethics. Consequently, the organization's focus is on the Jewish community. Its website includes endorsements from some of the leading rabbis in contemporary Orthodoxy. These rabbinic leaders not only praise the work of Renewal, but also explain how Renewal's work fits into the broader context of ethical Judaism.[2] Ultimately, donors and recipients alike acknowledge the fact that kidney donation does not just save the life of the recipient, but also positively impacts the lives of their family and friends. Parents live to love and raise their children, husbands and wives live to partake in the journey of life together, and friends live to share joy with each other and the world. Thanks to Renewal, hundreds of lives have been saved.

HODS

The Halachic Organ Donor Society: Shifting the Paradigm

I first met Robert (Robby) Berman when we were both in the thick of graduate school at Harvard University in the early aughts. I look back at my memories of Robby during that time with great affection. Whenever we interacted, I noted how smart, funny, and intensely passionate he was; even back then, he always strived to make the world a better place. He was driven, he was determined, he was talented; but most of all, Robby wanted to make a significant difference for the Jewish (and broader) community and was willing to be bold about it.

---

2. As explained elsewhere in this book, there is debate within the Jewish community regarding whether one should, or even may, donate their organs, in life or in death. See page *xx*. Renewal argues that virtually no *poseik* (decisor of Jewish law) forbids live donation, and it is oftentimes considered one of the highest of good deeds one can do as a fulfillment of *mitzvot* and religious duty.

In a previous life, Robby was a journalist and a comedian. But by the time I got to know him, he was already running the Halachic Organ Donor Society, known as HODS, which he founded in 2001. Even knowing the little about HODS I did in graduate school, I knew that this organization was special, unique, and a meaningful expression of the contemporary Jewish experience.

I got to know HODS further through my interactions with Robby. In 2006, during my rabbinical studies, I invited Robby to speak at the yeshiva where I was learning in Efrat. When I returned to the United States, I continued to invite him to different cities to give presentations about the work that HODS does every day to protect life while upholding the highest standards of Jewish legal thinking and ethics.

HODS' mission is simple: "To save lives by increasing organ donations from Jews to the general population (Jews and non-Jews alike)."[3] The organization focuses on educating people about organ donations, and the medical and *halachic* (Jewish law) considerations for it.[4] Its representatives have given thousands of lectures all over the world on topics related to organ donation, and have provided rabbinic consultation for Jews who may want to donate organs. The organization's website features content addressing what *halakhah* says about organ donation. As such, HODS works diligently to ensure that the decision to donate organs is based on fact and neither superstition nor mistaken religious considerations. HODS makes it easier for people who are skeptical (or unaware) of current trends

---

3. See https://hods.org.

4. HODS had helped facilitate the matching of a few living kidney donors and recipients, but eventually decided to focus exclusively on encouraging others to become donors after they die.

of Jewish legal thought to understand the issues, in the hope that they will find organ donation a viable option for them.

Part of HODS' work is normalizing attitudes toward organ donation. And one of the most brilliant tactics they have used is the donor card. The organization also offers a donor card that allows Jews to donate based on the specific *halachic* positions they may hold. One of the biggest issues regarding the *halachic* aspect of organ donation is the exact definition of death. There are several branches of thought on the matter, with some rabbinic authorities considering the cessation of cardiac activity along with brain death as death, while others maintain that brain death alone qualifies as death even if the heart continues to beat.[5] The organ donation card offered by HODS allows the donor to indicate which of the two definitions of death must be met so that their organs may be used.

Out of the 341 rabbis who carried HODS donor cards as of 2019, 85% define brain death with a beating heart as death; having the choice on the card helps a wider group of people feel comfortable signing up for an organ donor card. The ability to choose to donate organs after death is a positive step regardless of one's *halachic* position; but, at the same time, selecting the medically accepted brain death approach greatly expands the number of organs available for potential donation.

During my own journey with the organization, I found HODS' resources to be thorough, helpful, and theologically sound. While my type of donation didn't exactly apply, as it was a living donation, having a direct line to experts and deep thinkers on the matter was reassuring and helpful.

It's amazing to think that since its founding, HODS has helped save hundreds of lives. Robby and his team have fulfilled

---

5. Brain death is typically the medically standard definition; still, many religious leaders also require the cessation of heartbeat.

the Jewish mandate to save life at all costs thousands of times over. And there's so much more potential for them to further actualize their mission. Indeed, in addition to the rabbis registered with the organization, over two hundred physicians are also registered. But the intangible element of kindness matters just as much – kindness that brings strangers together in the shared vision of a repaired world. Just look at HODS' website, which features emotional testimonials from organ recipients of organs from Orthodox donors. As just one example, one man who waited a decade for a new liver stated that, had he not received the donation when he did, he most likely would not have been able to be a father to his children, born only three months later.

No matter where you stand on any technical questions about organ donation, the incredible gift that HODS contributes to the world cannot be denied. Robby and his team are among the holiest figures of this generation. The achievements of their work are awe-inspiring.

You can learn more by visiting the HODS website for a multitude of resources on the complexities and realities of organ donation. In addition, HODS offers speakers who can give presentations in your community. HODS provides brochures, web-based information for high school students, and a web-based quiz which allows readers to test their knowledge of organ donation and its concomitant *halachic* issues.

HODS shifted the paradigm for feelings about organ donation in contemporary Judaism. Now it is up to us to catch up to their point of view and become true allies in their cause. This organization continuously works to educate people on these issues, to recruit more and more people to register every day. Thanks to their tireless efforts, hundreds more people are getting a second chance at life. We should be honored to join with such an inspirational group of leaders.

Matnat Chayim
Matnat Chayim: Bringing the Gift of Life

In Hebrew, *matnat chayim* means "a gift of life." It is only fitting that an organization dedicated to kidney donation uses the phrase as both the name and creed of its mission. Matnat Chayim is an Israeli nonprofit whose goal is to encourage Israelis, particularly from the Orthodox Jewish community, to donate kidneys to those in need. Founded in 2009, the idea for Matnat Chayim was formed after a Jerusalem rabbi, Yeshayahu Heber, suddenly needed dialysis treatments. He was later saved by a kidney donation from a friend, but while on dialysis he met a young boy named Pinchas who desperately needed a kidney transplant. Rabbi Heber managed to find someone who agreed to donate to Pinchas, but the boy died before the operation could take place. In response to his tragic passing, Rabbi Heber formed Matnat Chayim to assist families in locating healthy donors for their loved ones who need transplants. Matnat Chayim began as a compassionate idea and has turned into a thriving, ever-growing and groundbreaking enterprise.

Matnat Chayim operates out of Israel and mainly supports kidney transplantation within the country, as international transplants are complex, and there are plenty of Israelis in need. In the years since its founding, Matnat Chayim has successfully helped facilitate more than a thousand kidney transplants, with many more planned in the coming years. The medical board of the organization is available for consultation for each case, to ensure that each party's needs are met. Matnat Chayim volunteers are available around the clock to provide support, guidance, and to answer any questions the donor or recipient may have regarding the transplant.

The Matnat Chayim website[6] offers a number of different

---

6. Learn more at kilya.org.il/en/. ("Kilya" means kidney in Hebrew.)

halachic opinions, as donors have a significant concern for religious considerations. The site answers specific religious questions which may not be answered elsewhere. The website also provides a wealth of information explaining the details of what kidney donation is, who can be a kidney donor, how to become a kidney donor, and what happens after donation. The site also features numerous testimonials from donors and recipients alike, all telling how their lives have been changed for the better as a result of the procedure.

Matnat Chayim offers no compensation for donation and receives no payment from transplant recipients. The organization makes clear that it in no way intends to pressure people to take action, but rather to provide information to those with the interest so they can make the best, most informed decision for themselves. The organization's primary goal is to help those in need get a second chance at life through donation. Israeli donors are compensated for lost work days, health insurance, transportation and other expenses by the government, so that donors can volunteer to save a life without facing economic hardship.

The Matnat Chayim website also features a page about children on dialysis, presenting dozens of Israeli children who receive this treatment and are in need of kidney transplants. This information underscores the fact that adults can, in fact, donate to children; Matnat Chayim has been involved in many of these successful transplants. As the founding of the organization was sparked by the tragic loss of a young boy's life, Matnat Chayim again and again achieves its goal of honoring the life and legacy of its inspiration.

In my interview with Judy Firestone Singer, Vice President of Resource Development for Matnat Chayim, which is included in this book, she mentioned to me that "Israel is a family-based society and everybody knows everybody." For her and the work of Matnat Chayim, this sentiment means that organ donation in Israel does not feel outside of one's everyday routine. Rather, people care for each other across the board, and organ donation is an expression of that universal love. Matnat Chayim provides an outlet for this love. And the world is all the better for it.

The Kidney Matchmaker
Chaya Lipschutz: A One-Stop Shop of Kidney Donation Advocacy

For years, Chaya Lipschutz has been known as one of the most indefatigable names for kidney donation advocacy in the Jewish community (and beyond). Since selflessly donating a kidney to a complete stranger in 2005, Chaya has worked tirelessly to ensure that more people receive kidneys from kindhearted donors; she also works to find suitable donors for liver transplants. When I learned about Chaya's story, I was instantly struck by the kindness she displayed through her altruistic donation. But it was her continuing journey that left an indelible impression on my own work in the field.

Most remarkably, Chaya's road to kidney donation began in the humblest of ways. While reading the newspaper, she saw an ad desperately seeking a donor for a kidney. Though the forum was unusual, Chaya responded with pure selflessness by answering the ad and saving someone's life. This was in September 2005.

The experience affected her deeply. After the donation was complete and Chaya was discharged from the hospital, she set up a booth at the Jewish Market Place Expo [in New York] to promote live kidney donation; this expo took place only three months after Chaya's surgery. In the months following her donation, Lipschutz was profiled by several media outlets, and her story reached across the world. She was deemed the

"Kidney Matchmaker" for her work matching donors with recipients (since then both her brother and nephew have also donated a kidney). She has spoken at many events and has been interviewed on television and radio programs about the work she is doing. She's received countless accolades for her work and was even proclaimed a Hometown Hero by New York State Assemblyman Dov Hikind.

To promote her work, Chaya created a website to provide potential donors and recipients easy access to information regarding donation and transplantation.[7] The website is a deep repository of inspirational stories, testimonials, and resources for those who are at all stages of their kidney donation journey, from those who are only starting to think about donating, to those wondering how to be advocates, to those who have followed through on the whole process. All the work Chaya does is on a volunteer basis. She never charges for her services and acts only as the "matchmaker" (as it were) to connect likely donors to vulnerable recipients. Her only hope is that people in need can find a donor and have their lives spared from years of misery and pain.

To date, Chaya has been remarkably successful at finding donors through a variety of platforms, including: online Jewish groups in America and Israel, craigslist, a radio program she was on, flyers she hung up for people in need of a kidney, social media, and people who found her through searches on the internet. At the same time, she's been contacted directly by people who found her website and were in desperate need of someone to turn to.

Although Chaya is an Orthodox Jew, her services do not discriminate: she aids and cares for people from all walks of life. Though her focus has always been the Jewish community, her

---

7. www.kidneymitzvah.com.

overall interest is finding suitable kidneys for as many people as possible. One of her kidney recipients who is not Jewish once told her, "I tell everyone that a Jewish person helped save my life." She continues to fight every day to further donation, as more and more people are added to the transplant list yearly.

To learn about the life and work of Chaya is a blessing. There are so many heroes who walk among us that they simply blend into the crowd. It's certainly an honor to write about Chaya's work and it gives me great comfort knowing that there is someone who is untiringly dedicated to ensuring that all those who are in desperate need of a life-saving kidney are one step closer to receiving one. The fact that Chaya is a one-stop shop for advocacy, comfort, and wisdom is a heartwarming reminder that it only takes one person to help heal this world. For, indeed, even just one person can make a world of difference; Chaya Lipschutz is proof of that.

Conclusion

Some years ago, crying, scared, but full of faith, I was wheeled away from my loving wife and into major surgery at The Mount Sinai Hospital as I had the great privilege of donating a kidney to a stranger. Since my procedure, I've learned so much more. Here are just 10 of the new deep lessons that I'm working to integrate more deeply into my life:

1. Strangers are merely those we haven't shared love with yet.
2. The Creator truly owns our bodies, which we only have on temporary loan. With this perspective, enjoying a luxury must give us serious pause when it's at the expense of another's life.
3. Lying vulnerable in a hospital bed and urinating into a bucket is a humbling reminder that health is a fleeting façade. There are only the sick & the not-yet-sick.
4. Philosophy matters, but developing a life philosophy really matters. If someone we love passes away, as difficult as it is in that moment, we are not desecrating their body by having the medical team remove their organs to save another's life. Rather, we are honoring their soul by giving them one last *mitzvah* to perform with their body. Those organs don't die with the body, but become eternal!

5. Go to the "inner place" where there are intense emotions. Where there is fear, there is often real opportunity.

6. The Satmar Hasidic Bikkur Cholim will ensure you gain weight after surgery with the most amazing (kosher vegan) peanut butter cookies that magically arrive every few minutes. It is almost worth having a major surgery just to get those holy Hasidic cookies.

7. I've taken far more from the world than I have given back. It requires radical interventions to break from our everyday routines of addressing our own needs. I fail miserably every hour of the day in trying to tip the scales toward being radically other-focused, but I must not stop trying.

8. Making a personal journey a public journey has its challenges, but also opens doors that need to be opened. I now have the blessing of dozens of new relationships with inspiring folks looking for support in their organ donation journey.

9. The opportunities to give are literally everywhere. If we truly embrace this as our life mission, then the invisible people become visible, the silent cries become heard, and our work in repairing the world can be increased a million-fold!

10. Having an amazing life partner enables one to live not only pragmatically but to dream.

There is so much for us all to do!

Thank you so much for reading and joining me on this very personal journey.

God bless you!

Contact List
of Organizations

For those considering donation, please feel free to reach out to me directly:

Rabbi Shmuly Yanklowitz

✉ RabbiYanklowitz@gmail.com

HODS

MISSION: To save lives by increasing organ donations from Jews to the general population (Jews and non-Jews alike).

⊕ https://hods.org/

☏ 212-213-5087

Renewal

MISSION: Renewal saves lives by helping facilitate kidney transplants for those suffering with chronic kidney disease. We provide guidance and support to help patients and their families navigate all the medical challenges of coping with their condition.

⊕ https://www.renewal.org/

☏ 718-431-9831

Matnat Chaim

MISSION: Matnat Chayim is an Israeli nonprofit dedicated to encouraging healthy volunteers to donate kidneys to patients who require a transplant. None of our kidney donors receive monetary compensation for their donation and most are altruistic donors who do not know their recipients prior to the procedure.

⊕ https://kilya.org.il/en/
✆ Outside of Israel: +972-50-377 9104
✆ Israel: 050-377 9104

Kidney Matchmaker

⊕ http://www.kidneymitzvah.com/
✉ kidneymitzvah@aol.com
✆ 917-627-8336

National Kidney Foundation

MISSION: The National Kidney Foundation is the leading organization in the U.S. dedicated to the awareness, prevention, and treatment of kidney disease for hundreds of thousands of healthcare professionals, millions of patients and their families, and tens of millions of Americans at risk.

⊕ https://www.kidney.org
✉ info@kidney.org
✆ 800-622-9010

American Kidney Fund

MISSION: To help people fight kidney disease and live healthier lives. We fulfill that mission by providing a complete spectrum of programs and services: prevention activities, top-rated health educational resources, and direct financial assistance enabling low-income U.S. dialysis and transplant patients to access lifesaving medical care.

⊕ http://www.kidneyfund.org
✆ 800-638-8299

National Kidney Registry

MISSION: The mission of the NKR is to save and improve the lives of people facing kidney failure by increasing the quality, speed and number of living donor transplants in the world as well as protecting all living kidney donors.

⊕ https://www.kidneyregistry.org/

United Network of Organ Sharing

MISSION: Unite and strengthen the donation and transplant community to save lives.

⊕ https://unos.org/

☏ 888-894-6361

Donate Life America

MISSION: To increase the number of donated organs, eyes, and tissues available to save and heal lives through transplantation while developing a culture where donation is embraced as a fundamental human responsibility.

⊕ https://www.donatelife.net

☏ 804-377-3580

American Transplant Foundation

MISSION: To save lives by reducing the growing list of women, men, and children who are waiting for a transplant.

⊕ https://www.americantransplantfoundation.org/

Living Kidney Donors Network

MISSION: To educate people in need of a kidney transplant about living donation and to prepare them to effectively communicate their need to family members and friends.

⊕ https://lkdn.org/

☏ 312-473-3772

American Society of Transplantation

MISSION: An organization dedicated to advancing the field of transplantation and improving patient care by promoting research, education, advocacy, organ donation, and service to the community.

🌐 https://www.myast.org/

📞 856-439-9986

Southwest Transplant Alliance

MISSION: To save lives through organ and tissue donation and transplantation.

🌐 https://www.organ.org/

📞 214-522-0255

Transplant First Academy

MISSION: To inspire a life-saving alternative to our nation's life-threatening wait for a kidney.

🌐 https://transplantfirst.org/

Reach Kidney Care

MISSION: To improve the health of all people with kidney disease every day.

🌐 https://www.reachkidneycare.org/

📞 833-447-4397

The Living Bank

MISSION: To advance living organ donation to confront the shortage of organs needed for life-saving transplants.

🌐 https://www.livingbank.org

📞 800-528-2971

National Living Donor Assistance Center

MISSION: To reduce the financial disincentives to living organ donation.

🌐 https://www.livingdonorassistance.org/

📞 888-870-5002

Alliance for Paired Kidney Donation

MISSION: To save lives by securing a living donor kidney transplant for every patient who needs one.

⊕ https://paireddonation.org/

☎ 419-740-5249

Kidney Donation Online Discussion Forums

Some Facebook Groups:

Living Donor Support Group-only donors & those considering donation

Kidney Support: Dialysis, Transplants, Donors and Recipients

Living Kidney Donors Support Group

Kidney Transplant Recipients & Donors

Transplant Talk

Living Donors Online!

Organ Transplant – Living Donor Awareness Group

Living Kidney Donors Network

Kidney Donor Conversations

Living kidney donors

Other Online Groups:

LIVING DONORS ONLINE:
https://livingdonorsonline.org/ldosmf/index.php

NKF PEERS:
https://www.kidney.org/patients/peers

ORGAN TRANSPLANT SUPPORT:
https://www.organtransplantsupport.org/

About the Author

Rabbi Yanklowitz has twice been named one of America's Top Rabbis by *Newsweek* and has been named by *The Forward* as one of the 50 most influential Jews and one of the most inspiring rabbis in America. Rabbi Yanklowitz is the author of over twenty books on Jewish ethics. His writings have appeared in outlets as diverse as *The New York Times, The Wall Street Journal, The Washington Post, The Guardian,* and *The Atlantic,* among many other secular and religious publications. He has served as speaker at the World Economic Forum in Davos, Switzerland, and as a Rothschild Fellow in Cambridge, UK.

Rav Shmuly received a Masters from Harvard University and a Doctorate from Columbia University. He serves as the President & Dean of Valley Beit Midrash (a global center for learning and action); is the Founder & President of Uri L'Tzedek (the Orthodox Social Justice movement); is the Founder and President of Shamayim (Jewish animal advocacy); and the Founder and President of YATOM (Jewish foster and adoption network). Rabbi Shmuly, his wife Shoshana, and their four children live in Scottsdale, Arizona. They are also foster parents.

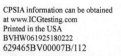